STUDY GUIDE TO PERSONALITY DISORDERS

A Companion to
The American Psychiatric Publishing Textbook of Personality Disorders,
Second Edition

STUDY GUIDE TO PERSONALITY DISORDERS

A Companion to
The American Psychiatric Publishing Textbook of Personality Disorders,
Second Edition

Edited by

Philip R. Muskin, M.D.

Professor of Psychiatry,
Columbia University Medical Center;
Chief, Consultation-Liaison Psychiatry,
New York–Presbyterian Hospital/Columbia Campus;
Faculty, Columbia University Center for Psychoanalytic
Training and Research, New York, New York

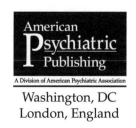

American **P**sychiatric Publishing
A Division of American Psychiatric Association

Washington, DC
London, England

Copyright © 2015 American Psychiatric Association
ALL RIGHTS RESERVED

Manufactured in the United States of America on acid-free paper
18 17 16 15 14   5 4 3 2 1
ISBN 978-1-58562-499-7
First Edition

Typeset in Adobe's Palatino LT Std and Helvetica LT Std

American Psychiatric Publishing
A Division of American Psychiatric Association
1000 Wilson Boulevard
Arlington, VA 22209-3901
www.appi.org

Contents

Contributors ix

Preface xiii

Part I: Questions

CHAPTER 1
Personality Disorders: Recent History and New Directions 3

CHAPTER 2
Theories of Personality and Personality Disorders. 6

CHAPTER 3
Articulating a Core Dimension of Personality Pathology 9

CHAPTER 4
Development, Attachment, and Childhood Experiences 12

CHAPTER 5
Genetics and Neurobiology 15

CHAPTER 6
Prevalence, Sociodemographics, and Functional Impairment. 20

CHAPTER 7
Manifestations, Assessment, and Differential Diagnosis 23

CHAPTER 8
Course and Outcome 26

CHAPTER 9
Therapeutic Alliance. 29

CHAPTER 10
Psychodynamic Psychotherapies and Psychoanalysis 32

CHAPTER 11
Cognitive-Behavioral Therapy I: Basics and Principles 36

CHAPTER 12
Cognitive-Behavioral Therapy II:
Specific Strategies for Personality Disorders 39

CHAPTER 13
Group, Family, and Couples Therapies.............................42

CHAPTER 14
Psychoeducation 45

CHAPTER 15
Somatic Treatments..48

CHAPTER 16
Collaborative Treatment..51

CHAPTER 17
Boundary Issues...54

CHAPTER 18
Assessing and Managing Suicide Risk.............................57

CHAPTER 19
Substance Use Disorders...60

CHAPTER 20
Antisocial Personality Disorder and Other Antisocial Behavior.........63

CHAPTER 21
Personality Disorders in the Medical Setting 66

CHAPTER 22
Personality Disorders in the Military Operational Environment 69

CHAPTER 23
Translational Research in Borderline Personality Disorder 72

CHAPTER 24
An Alternative Model for Personality Disorders
    DSM-5 SECTION III AND BEYOND.................................75

Part II: Answer Guide

CHAPTER 1
Personality Disorders: Recent History and New Directions.............81

CHAPTER 2
Theories of Personality and Personality Disorders...................87

CHAPTER 3
Articulating a Core Dimension of Personality Pathology 95

CHAPTER 4
Development, Attachment, and Childhood Experiences 100

CHAPTER 5
Genetics and Neurobiology 106

CHAPTER 6
Prevalence, Sociodemographics, and Functional Impairment. 119

CHAPTER 7
Manifestations, Assessment, and Differential Diagnosis 125

CHAPTER 8
Course and Outcome 131

CHAPTER 9
Therapeutic Alliance. 138

CHAPTER 10
Psychodynamic Psychotherapies and Psychoanalysis 144

CHAPTER 11
Cognitive-Behavioral Therapy I: Basics and Principles 152

CHAPTER 12
Cognitive-Behavioral Therapy II:
Specific Strategies for Personality Disorders 160

CHAPTER 13
Group, Family, and Couples Therapies. 167

CHAPTER 14
Psychoeducation 172

CHAPTER 15
Somatic Treatments 179

CHAPTER 16
Collaborative Treatment. 184

CHAPTER 17
Boundary Issues. 190

CHAPTER 18
Assessing and Managing Suicide Risk 197

CHAPTER 19
Substance Use Disorders. 206

CHAPTER 20
Antisocial Personality Disorder and Other Antisocial Behavior 212

CHAPTER 21
Personality Disorders in the Medical Setting 220

CHAPTER 22
Personality Disorders in the Military Operational Environment 229

CHAPTER 23
Translational Research in Borderline Personality Disorder 237

CHAPTER 24
An Alternative Model for Personality Disorders
 DSM-5 SECTION III AND BEYOND. 243

Contributors

Marra G. Ackerman, M.D.
Fellow, Psychosomatic Medicine, Department of Psychiatry Consultation-Liaison Service, New York-Presbyterian Hospital/Columbia University Medical Center, New York, New York

Iqbal "Ike" Ahmed, M.D.
Faculty Psychiatrist, Tripler Army Medical Center; Clinical Professor of Psychiatry, Uniformed Services University of Health Sciences; Clinical Professor of Psychiatry and Geriatric Medicine, University of Hawaii, Honolulu, Hawaii

Lawrence Amsel, M.D., M.P.H.
Assistant Professor of Clinical Psychiatry, Columbia University Medical Center, New York, New York

Robert J. Boland, M.D.
Professor of Psychiatry and Human Behavior, Alpert Medical School, Brown University, Providence, Rhode Island

Rachel Anne Caravella, M.D.
Fellow, Psychosomatic Medicine, Department of Psychiatry Consultation-Liaison Service, New York-Presbyterian Hospital/Columbia University Medical Center, New York, New York

Josepha A. Cheong, M.D.
Professor of Psychiatry, University of Florida College of Medicine, Gainesville, Florida; Assistant Chief, Psychiatry Section, Veterans Health Administration VISN 9, Nashville, Tennessee

Kelly L. Cozza, M.D., DFAPA, FAPM
Associate Professor, Department of Psychiatry, Uniformed Services University; Consultant, Department of Psychiatry, Walter Reed National Military Medical Center, Bethesda, Maryland

Meena Dasari, Ph.D.
Clinical Psychologist and Assistant Professor, New York University School of Medicine, New York, New York

Anna L. Dickerman, M.D.
Assistant Professor of Psychiatry, Weill Cornell Medical College; Assistant Attending Psychiatrist, Psychiatry Consultation-Liaison Service, New York-Presbyterian Hospital/Weill Cornell Medical Center, New York, New York

Nika Dyakina, D.O.
Assistant Professor of Psychiatry, Columbia University Medical Center; Associate Director of Pediatric Psychiatry Emergency and Consultation Services, Morgan Stanley Children's Hospital of New York, New York

Emily D. Gastelum, M.D.
Candidate, Columbia University Center for Psychoanalytic Training and Research; Instructor of Clinical Psychiatry at Columbia University Medical Center, New York State Psychiatric Institute, New York, New York

Adam Goldyne, M.D.
Associate Clinical Professor of Psychiatry, University of California San Francisco; Faculty, San Francisco Center for Psychoanalysis, San Francisco, California

Richard G. Hersh, M.D.
Associate Professor of Psychiatry, Columbia University Medical Center, New York, New York

Yael Holoshitz, M.D.
Fellow, Public Psychiatry Program, Columbia Psychiatry/New York State Psychiatric Institute, New York, New York

Sherry Katz-Bearnot, M.D.
Assistant Clinical Professor of Psychiatry, Columbia University Medical Center; Faculty, Columbia University Center for Psychoanalytic Training and Research, New York, New York

Sarah Richards Kim, M.D.
Fellow, Child and Adolescent Psychiatry, New York-Presbyterian Hospital/Weill Cornell Medical Center, New York, New York

John Luo, M.D.
Senior Physician Informaticist, UCLA Health; Professor of Clinical Psychiatry, David Geffen School of Medicine, UCLA, Los Angeles, California

Philip R. Muskin, M.D., M.A.
Professor of Psychiatry, Columbia University Medical Center; Chief, Consultation-Liaison Psychiatry, New York-Presbyterian Hospital/Columbia Campus; Faculty, Columbia University Center for Psychoanalytic Training and Research, New York, New York

Michelle Riba, M.D., M.S.
Professor and Associate Chair for Integrated Medical and Psychiatric Services, Department of Psychiatry, University of Michigan, Ann Arbor, Michigan

Lisa S. Seyfried, M.D.
Assistant Professor, Department of Psychiatry; Section Director, Psychiatry Hospital Services, University of Michigan, Ann Arbor, Michigan

David Steinberg, M.D.
Clinical Associate Professor of Psychiatry and Behavioral Health, Director of Education, Child and Adolescent Psychiatry, New York Medical College, Valhalla, New York

Wendy L. Thompson, M.D.
Professor of Clinical Psychiatry, Vice Chair for Education, Department of Psychiatry and Behavioral Science, New York Medical College, Valhalla, New York

Thomas E. Ungar M.D., M.Ed., CCFP, FCFP, FRCPC, DABPN
Associate Professor, University of Toronto; Chief of Psychiatry and Chief of Staff, North York General Hospital, Toronto, Ontario, Canada

Marcia L. Verduin, M.D.
Associate Dean for Students, Associate Professor of Psychiatry, University of Central Florida College of Medicine, Orlando, Florida

Disclosure of Interests

None of the contributors to this book have indicated competing interests to disclose during the year preceding manuscript submission.

Preface

This self-examination guide is a companion to, not a replacement of, reading *The American Psychiatric Publishing Textbook of Personality Disorders*. Patients with personality disorders can present diagnostic and therapeutic challenges. The textbook will prepare readers to understand the epidemiology, neurobiology, psychology, and treatment of patients with personality disorders. Therefore, we have attempted to organize questions along those domains. As you work through this self-examination book, let it guide you to chapters in the textbook as a path to your self-education. Some questions will seem obvious or easy, and some questions will be quite difficult. We have endeavored to use the style of question writing found in certification examinations; however, this is not a board preparation book. The contributors to this book are a group of clinicians and educators with a broad range of experience and expertise who undertook the task of writing the questions. The contributors have graciously donated the proceeds from this book to a charitable foundation.

Philip R. Muskin, M.D., Editor

Part I

Questions

CHAPTER 1

Personality Disorders: Recent History and New Directions

1.1 In the Collaborative Longitudinal Personality Disorders Study (CLPS), what percentage of patients meeting criteria for borderline personality disorder (BPD) at intake showed remission at 10-year follow-up?

A. 15%.
B. 35%.
C. 50%.
D. 65%.
E. 85%.

1.2 The second edition of the DSM aimed to introduce what major diagnostic concept to the way that PDs were conceptualized and described?

A. Diagnoses aimed to capture constellations of personality that were observable, measurable, enduring, and consistent over time.
B. Diagnoses made based on degree of social and occupational dysfunction.
C. Diagnoses reflected evolving and controversial psychoanalytic theories of the time.
D. Diagnoses focused on etiology and pathogenesis of symptoms.
E. Diagnoses clarified degree to which symptoms caused emotional suffering.

1.3 In DSM-III, what characteristic difference was thought to exist between Axis I and Axis II disorders, which allowed for the separation of the PDs from many other psychiatric illnesses?

A. Axis II disorders were thought to be less severe than Axis I disorders.
B. Axis II disorders were thought to be less genetically determined than Axis I disorders.
C. Axis II disorders were composed of persistent conditions versus the episodic disorders of Axis I.

D. Axis II disorders were derived from psychoanalytic theory, whereas Axis I disorders were empirically based.

E. Axis II disorders were thought to respond to therapy, whereas Axis I disorders were thought to respond to medications.

1.4 In the transition from DSM-II to DSM-III, schizoid PD was subcategorized into which three PDs?

A. Schizoid, schizotypal, passive-aggressive.
B. Schizoid, schizotypal, avoidant.
C. Schizotypal, borderline, avoidant.
D. Schizotypal, borderline, narcissistic.
E. Schizoid, narcissistic, passive-aggressive.

1.5 In the first edition of DSM, what clinical picture did "personality pattern disturbances" describe?

A. Innate, genetically based features of personality that are present from birth.
B. Conditions that in the absence of stress were not particularly pervasive and disabling.
C. Entrenched conditions likely to be recalcitrant to change.
D. Social deviance behaviors such as sexual deviations, addictions, and antisocial reaction.
E. Episodic personality changes due to mood and psychotic episodes.

1.6 In DSM-III, the work of multiple scholars of personality and emotional disturbances significantly influenced and shaped the emergence of what two PD descriptions?

A. Borderline and narcissistic.
B. Borderline and histrionic.
C. Narcissistic and schizotypal.
D. Histrionic and antisocial.
E. Schizotypal and antisocial.

1.7 Substantiated, evidence-based treatment guidelines exist for which of the following PDs?

A. Histrionic PD.
B. Paranoid PD.
C. Schizoid PD.
D. Antisocial PD.
E. BPD.

1.8 Reflecting the ongoing debate regarding how to conceptualize, understand, and thus adequately treat PDs, Section III of DSM-5 establishes a hybrid of what two models of diagnoses and classification?

A. Psychological and biological.
B. Cognitive and behavioral.
C. Dimensional and categorical.
D. State and trait.
E. Interpersonal and intrapersonal.

1.9 The organization of PDs into clusters, odd or eccentric; dramatic, emotional, or erratic; and anxious or fearful, reflects what type of diagnostic classification?

A. Etiological.
B. Dimensional.
C. Categorical.
D. Hierarchical.
E. Ontogenetic.

CHAPTER 2

Theories of Personality and Personality Disorders

2.1   Which of the following correctly describes the trait psychological model of personality disorders (PDs)?

   A. Trait psychology focuses less than psychodynamic or cognitive-social approaches on personality processes or functions.
   B. Trait psychology dichotomizes the pathological and the normal.
   C. Trait models define a personality disposition separate from a behavioral tendency.
   D. The trait model only incorporates psychodynamic and not biological theory.
   E. Trait models of PDs cannot be used to describe clinically derived categories.

2.2   What is a key feature of Cloninger's neurobiological model of personality?

   A. It divides personality structure into the two domains of temperament and character.
   B. It is based on findings from magnetic resonance imaging (MRI) studies.
   C. The model does not include a spiritual dimension.
   D. The model does not address modes of learning.
   E. It defines impulsivity as the major determinant of the presence or absence of PD.

2.3   Which idea listed below is a key feature of a psychodynamic point of view of PD?

   A. Personality disorders reflect specific pathological symptoms rather than constellations of psychological processes.
   B. Personality disorders are the result of the internalization of the attitudes of hostile, abusive, critical, or inconsistent parents and/or significant caretakers.
   C. Personality disorders are restricted to a single personality domain.
   D. Using the ego psychology model, patients with PDs consistently act in the best interests of others.
   E. Patients with PDs can weather momentary failures in the professional arena.

2.4 Which of the following statements is identified as a feature of the framework of Kernberg's psychodynamic theory of personality and PD?

A. Reality testing is not an important concern.
B. Borderline PD (BPD) in the DSM-5 is equivalent to borderline personality organization as described by Kernberg.
C. More severe personality structure is distinguished by more maladaptive modes of regulating emotions through immature, reality-distorting defenses.
D. Personality-disordered patients are able to generate multifaceted representations of themselves and significant others.
E. The conscious self-representations of narcissistic patients are not grandiose, although the ideal representations are grandiose.

2.5 What is a key feature of cognitive-social theories of PDs?

A. They are based on the idea that learned behaviors are generalized.
B. They assume that personality comprises relatively discrete learned processes that are not situation specific.
C. They do not include skills and competencies.
D. They do not take into account the role of environment but rather favor inherent traits and early life experience in the development of PDs.
E. They include the idea that problems in self-regulation are of particular relevance to severe PDs.

2.6 Which of the following is a key element in Linehan's concept of BPD?

A. In contrast to psychodynamic theories, it is silent on the importance of the development of a stable sense of self.
B. It downplays the importance of physiological responses to emotional arousal.
C. It defines a major problem in BPD as a difficulty in inhibiting inappropriate behavior related to intense affect.
D. It considers refocusing of attention as a maladaptive defense mechanism.
E. It downplays the importance of developing interpersonal strategies to the setting of personal goals.

2.7 Which of the options below correctly describes a feature of Westen's model of domains of personality functioning?

A. It is based on psychoanalytic theory but not on empirical research.
B. It is a trait model.
C. It requires the use of the Shedler-Westen Assessment Procedure (SWAP-200).
D. It uses insights drawn from many psychoanalytic theoretical schools of thought, including those of ego psychology, self psychology, attachment theory, and object relations theory.
E. It only describes disturbed personality styles and dynamics not healthy personality styles.

2.8 Benjamin's interpersonal theory of personality is called the Structural Analysis of Social Behavior (SASB). Which of the statements below is a correct description of the model?

A. The SASB is a one-dimensional model.
B. It is a circumflex model in which all three surfaces describe interpersonal patterns.
C. It is a model capable of specifying the interpersonal antecedents that elicit a patient's responses.
D. It is a model that aims to specify a single motivation to explain a behavior.
E. It is unrelated to the PD diagnoses as described in the DSM.

2.9 Which statement below correctly describes the utility of behavioral genetic approaches to PDs?

A. They address the lack of consensus among trait psychologists regarding which traits to study by studying the causes of trait covariation.
B. They preferentially study abnormal personality traits found in PDs rather than normal personality traits.
C. They direct twin and adoption studies that demonstrate consistent and precise heritability of PDs.
D. They demonstrate that the heritability of PDs is less than 20%.
E. They show that BPD is primarily biologically determined.

2.10 Early maladaptive schemas (EMSs) are an augmentation of cognitive-behavioral personality theory promulgated by Young to address aspects of personality development, which take place at a young age. Which statement about EMS below is correct?

A. It is an extension of Kohut's theories of the grandiose self.
B. Young believes that schema maintenance, schema avoidance, and schema compensation are the three most important cognitive processes involving schemas that define key features of PDs.
C. Young's theories are incompatible with psychodynamic and attachment theories.
D. EMSs equate with automatic thoughts and underlying assumptions.
E. Young has identified 10 EMSs.

Articulating a Core Dimension of Personality Pathology

3.1 The DSM-5 Personality and Personality Disorders Work Group proposed that core impairments found in personality disorders (PDs) should be assessed using a dimensional approach. Which of the following clinicians might have disagreed with using a dimensional approach to assessing psychopathology?

A. Sir Francis Galton.
B. Emil Kraepelin.
C. Otto Kernberg.
D. Jean Piaget.
E. J.C. Prichard.

3.2 A number of reliable and valid measures exist for assessing personality functioning and psychopathology. Which of the following measures provides a dimensional assessment of identity, primitive defenses, and reality testing and is based upon a model of personality advanced by Kernberg?

A. General Assessment of Personality Disorder (GAPD).
B. Severity Indices of Personality Problems (SIPP).
C. Social Cognition and Object Relations Scale (SCORS).
D. Structured Interview of Personality Organization (STIPO).
E. Thematic Apperception Test (TAT).

3.3 In the literature review conducted by Bender et al. (2011), which of the following rubrics captured components most central to effective personality functioning?

A. Identity, self-direction, empathy, intimacy.
B. Reality testing, defensive structure, object representations, self representations.
C. Cognition, libido, affective lability, impulse control.
D. Obsessionality, hysteria, masochism, narcissism.
E. Mood, anxiety, psychosis, substance use.

3.4 Mary meets seven of nine criteria for borderline PD (BPD), whereas Andrea meets five of nine criteria for BPD. Which of the following is likely to be a true statement about each person?

   A. Andrea is more likely than Mary to meet criteria for additional PDs.
   B. Mary is more likely than Andrea to meet criteria for additional PDs.
   C. Andrea is more likely than Mary to have a history of childhood trauma.
   D. Mary is more likely than Andrea to have a history of childhood trauma.
   E. There is not any meaningful difference between Mary and Andrea's likelihood of comorbidity or history of trauma.

3.5 The Level of Personality Functioning Scale (LPFS; American Psychiatric Association, 2013) represents a single-item composite evaluation of impairment in identity, self-direction, empathy, and intimacy. It was designed to serve as a basis for determining global level of impairment in personality functioning in DSM-5. Which of the following is true of the LPFS?

   A. It has good sensitivity and good specificity for identifying the presence or absence of DSM-IV PDs.
   B. It has good sensitivity but poor specificity for identifying the presence or absence of DSM-IV PDs.
   C. It has poor sensitivity but good specificity for identifying the presence or absence of DSM-IV PDs.
   D. It has poor sensitivity and poor specificity for identifying the presence or absence of DSM-IV PDs.

3.6 In which of the following areas did specific PD diagnoses prove useful as a supplement to the LPFS rating of personality impairment?

   A. Estimated prognosis.
   B. Estimating number of medical comorbidities.
   C. Optimal level of treatment intensity.
   D. Psychosocial functioning.
   E. Risk assessment.

3.7 Morey et al. (2013) demonstrated that clinicians felt the clinical utility of DSM-IV criteria was more useful than the DSM-5 LPFS rating scale for which of the following?

   A. Communicating to the patient.
   B. Communication with other professionals.
   C. Patient description.
   D. Research studies.
   E. Treatment planning.

3.8   Reliable and valid clinician-administered measures of personality functioning and psychopathology generally have a significant focus on which of the following?

   A. Affective lability.
   B. IQ scores.
   C. History of traumatic life events.
   D. Representations of self and other.
   E. Reality testing and perceptual disturbances.

CHAPTER 4

Development, Attachment, and Childhood Experiences

4.1   Who formulated the basic tenets of the attachment theory?

    A. Mary Ainsworth.
    B. John Bowlby.
    C. Carol George.
    D. Anthony Bateman and Peter Fonagy.
    E. Jean Piaget.

4.2   A child is playing in the room and does not react when the mother leaves the room or when a stranger enters. The child continues to play when the mother returns. The description of this "Strange Situation" is most consistent with which of the following attachment pattern in infants?

    A. Anxious/resistant.
    B. Securely attached.
    C. Disoriented/disorganized.
    D. Anxious/preoccupied.
    E. Avoidant.

4.3   What is the correlation between infant attachment predicted by the Strange Situation procedure and adult attachment classification based on the AAI?

    A. 68%–75%.
    B. 5%–15%.
    C. 100%.
    D. 20%–35%.
    E. 75%–90%.

4.4 Childhood trauma is strongly associated with which of the following personality disorder (PD) and adult attachment style pairs?

A. Schizoid PD and incoherent/disorganized.
B. Borderline PD (BPD) and incoherent/disorganized.
C. Dependent PD and anxious/preoccupied.
D. Antisocial PD and avoidant/ dismissing.
E. Histrionic PD and anxious/preoccupied.

4.5 In addition to oxytocin, which other neurotransmitter has been shown to play a crucial role in attachment behavior?

A. Serotonin.
B. Anandamide.
C. Dopamine.
D. Substance P.
E. Glutamine.

4.6 What is the effect of oxytocin in the insecurely attached patient with BPD?

A. It increases trust and reduces dysphoric response to social stress.
B. It increases trust but increases dysphoric response to social stress.
C. It does not have any effect on trust in individuals with BPD.
D. It decreases trust but reduces dysphoric response to social stress.
E. It decreases trust and increases dysphoric response to social stress.

4.7 Which of the following is not a key determinant in problematic affect regulation and self-control stemming from dysfunctional attachment relationship?

A. A robust mentalizing capacity.
B. Maltreatment.
C. Failure to develop good interpersonal skills.
D. Failure to self-reflect.
E. High levels of parental mentalization about their children.

4.8 Mind-related comments by mothers when a child was 6 months predicted what capacity of the child at 45 and 48 months?

A. IQ scores.
B. Vocabulary.
C. Secure attachment.
D. Imaginary play.
E. Mentalizing.

4.9   What aspect of child development is explained by the theory of pedagogy?

   A. School readiness.
   B. Attachment.
   C. Tantrums.
   D. Subjectivity.
   E. Pretend play.

4.10   Which two adult attachment styles are associated with treatment dropout?

   A. Secure and avoidant.
   B. Secure and preoccupied.
   C. Anxious and disorganized.
   D. Avoidant and preoccupied.
   E. Secure and disorganized.

4.11   In a randomized controlled trial of transference-focused psychotherapy (TFP), dialectical behavior therapy (DBT), and supportive therapy, which treatment modality achieved an increased number of patients classified as secure after treatment?

   A. Treatment as usual.
   B. TFP.
   C. DBT.
   D. Supportive therapy.
   E. Treatment has no effect on attachment.

CHAPTER 5

Genetics and Neurobiology

5.1 DSM-5 conceptualizes personality disorders (PDs) in terms of which of the following assessment systems?

A. Dimensional approach.
B. Interacting traits approach.
C. Categorical classification.
D. Interpersonal functioning scale.
E. Impairment-based metrics.

5.2 Affective instability, a defining trait of borderline PD (BPD), is associated with changes *primarily* in which of the following affects?

A. Anger, jealousy, shame.
B. Anger, euphoria, guilt.
C. Anger, anxiety, depression.
D. Anger, suspicion, distrust.
E. Anger, disappointment, loneliness.

5.3 Which of the following is an empirical finding supporting the notion of heightened sensitivity to emotional stimuli in patients with BPD?

A. A bias to preferentially identify faces with negative or hostile emotions.
B. A need for greater visual information than control subjects.
C. Greater capacity for reallocation of attention than control subjects when faced with affective stimuli.
D. Greater capacity for cognitive reappraisal than control subjects when faced with affective stimuli.
E. Greater reliance on habituation to control highly charged stimuli.

5.4 In healthy people, certain brain regions have been paired with particular functions and thus have become regions of interest for assessing PD and other psychopathology. Which of the following is an empirically based pairing of regions and their primary functionality?

A. Rostral anterior cingulate cortex (ACC) and cognitive processing.
B. Insula and motor coordination.

C. Fusiform gyrus and facial recognition.
D. Amygdala and decision making.
E. Dorsal ACC and visual processing.

5.5 Brain volumes of specific regions, as measured by magnetic resonance imaging (MRI), have shown differences between patients with BPD and healthy control subjects. Which of the following is a consistently reported difference between patients with BPD and healthy control subjects?

A. Smaller amygdala volumes in patients with BPD.
B. Decreased cingulate gray matter volumes in patients with BPD.
C. Decreased anterior cingulate gray matter volumes in female patients with BPD.
D. Increased hippocampus volumes in patients with BPD.
E. Decreased ventral cingulate volumes in patients with BPD, independent of co-morbid depression.

5.6 Difficulties with emotion regulation in patients with BPD have long been recognized. Which of the following is an empirically supported functional MRI (fMRI) finding that supports this clinical observation?

A. Compared with healthy control subjects, patients with BPD showed greater activation of dorsal ACC and intraparietal sulcus in response to attempts to downregulate their responses to disturbing pictures.
B. Compared with healthy control subjects, patients with BPD showed less fusiform face region activity when viewing photographs depicting emotional faces.
C. Compared with healthy control subjects, patients with BPD showed rapid behavioral habituation to negative pictures.
D. Compared with healthy control subjects, patients with BPD showed greater activation of the primary visual areas and the superior temporal gyrus when viewing negative versus neutral pictures.
E. Compared with healthy control subjects, patients with BPD showed a decrease in insular and an increase in orbitofrontal cortex (OFC) activity during attempted distancing.

5.7 Which of the following symptom domains is *least* accounted for by genetic factors?

A. Affective instability.
B. Identity problems.
C. Negative relationships.
D. Avoidance.
E. Self-harm.

5.8 Impulsive aggression plays an important role in the clinical presentation of patients with BPD. Which of the following is true regarding the nature and measurement of this aggression?

A. Self-reported impulsive aggression remains the best way to distinguish BPD from PD.
B. The Point Subtraction Aggression Paradigm (PSAP) is an effective behavioral measure of impulsive-aggressive tendencies.
C. Subjects with high impulsive aggression also showed greater OFC activity during a provocation.
D. Impulsive aggression is measurable under both provoking and nonprovoking situations.
E. Impulsive aggression is mostly confined to BPD, being a rare manifestation of another PD.

5.9 Impulsive aggression in BPD has been shown to have neurobiological correlates. Which of the following is a neurobiological correlate of impulsive aggression in BPD?

A. Increased metabolism from serotonergic stimulation with D,L-fenfluramine.
B. Increased synthesis of serotonin under normal resting conditions.
C. Adult-onset lesions of the OFC.
D. Disruption of coupling of the OFC and the amygdala.
E. Increased brain metabolism in OFC and anterior cingulate gyrus (ACG) in response to meta-chlorophenylpiperazine (mCPP) administration.

5.10 The trust game is a laboratory simulation game that measures "players'" capacity for interpersonal trust. Choose the most accurate statement about the findings on patients with BPD versus healthy control subjects using this laboratory task.

A. Consistent with rapid overvaluation of others, patients with BPD self-reported greater trust in game partners.
B. When playing the trustee role, patients with BPD induced distrust in healthy control game partners.
C. Consistent with interpersonal sensitivity, the anterior insula of patients with BPD demonstrated greater responsivity (than healthy control subjects) to the amount of trust shown toward them.
D. Patients with BPD tended to underestimate the potential of being taken advantage of in the game.
E. Despite interpersonal difficulties, the patients with BPD did not become hypervigilant to being taken advantage of in the game.

5.11   Which of the following therapies is least likely to treat successfully the interpersonal hypersensitivity associated with patients with BPD?

A. Mentalization-based therapy.
B. Facial emotion-recognition training.
C. Social norm violation awareness training.
D. Desensitization to perceived rejection.
E. Motivational interviewing.

5.12   Pain perception in patients with BPD has long been recognized to be anomalous and to be related to self-injurious behaviors. Choose the answer that most correctly pairs an fMRI finding and its clinical correlate.

A. Patients with BPD showed decreased activation of the dorsolateral prefrontal cortex in response to pain and experienced pain as less aversive.
B. Thermal stimuli, acting as an emotional distracter, reduced amygdala response to emotional pictures in patients with BPD but not in healthy control subjects.
C. Patients with BPD showed less signal decrease than healthy control subjects in posterior aspect of the default mode network (DMN) during pain processing, indicating greater self-preoccupation and less aversive experience of the pain.
D. ACC and right amygdala were unchanged in patients with BPD during pain processing, indicating a decreased pain response.
E. Greater connectivity in the DMN system in patients with BPD indicates they overengage emotional regulatory systems.

5.13   Schizotypal PD (STPD) is characterized by disturbances of many areas including cognition. Choose the statement that most accurately describes the cognitive and associated deficits in STPD.

A. Cognitive deficits in patients with STPD have similar severity to those found in schizophrenia.
B. Auditory but not visual memory deficits have been found in patients with STPD.
C. Smooth pursuit eye movement deficits have been identified in patients with STPD.
D. Failure of medial frontal pole and anterior frontal pole to compensate for frontal lobe deficits may explain cognitive symptoms in patients with STPD.
E. P_{50} auditory-evoked potential abnormalities have been shown to differentiate schizophrenia patients from patients with STPD.

5.14   Symptoms profiles in patients with STPD are correlated with neurobiological findings. Choose the correct statement regarding the association of neurobiological findings and symptoms profiles in patients with STPD.

A. Negative and positive symptoms of STPD are both associated with increased dopamine activity and reversed with dopamine antagonists.
B. Patients with STPD are better buffered than patients with schizophrenia in regard to subcortical dopamine release provoked by $[^{123}I]$iodobenzamide (IBZM).

C. Positron emission tomography (PET) studies indicate a decrease in D_1 receptor availability in STPD, suggesting a mechanism for amphetamine administration in improving the associated cognitive deficits.

D. D_1 antagonists may enhance cognition in patients with STPD by lowering the excess dopamine activity in the frontal lobes.

E. The fact that neuroleptics have failed to have an effect on psychotic-like symptoms of STPD has been explained by the negative effects that blocking dopamine activity in these patients may have.

5.15   Social function is impaired in patients with STPD. Choose the correct statement regarding social deficits in patients with STPD.

A. Social anxiety is not qualitatively distinct from the social anxiety in other PDs.

B. Smooth pursuit eye movement deficits correlate with social difficulties in healthy control subjects.

C. Facial emotion-cognition failed to correlate with social anxiety in healthy control subjects.

D. The social anxiety of a patient with STPD will attenuate as he or she becomes familiar with particular individuals or social situations.

E. Patients with STPD report concerns that they will be rejected as the driving cognition behind their anxiety.

5.16   Antisocial PD (ASPD) and psychopathy have long been recognized as different but overlapping concepts. Choose the correct statement regarding differences between these conditions.

A. Psychopaths show greater difficulty identifying fear in facial emotion tasks than patients with ASPD.

B. On an emotional version of a go/no-go task, patients with psychopathy showed blunted processing of negative emotional words, whereas patients with ASPD showed appropriate processing of negative emotional words regardless of inhibitory control demands.

C. Both patients with psychopathy and patients with ASPD demonstrate aggression of the instrumental (strategic) type.

D. Executive functioning, which is responsible for behavioral control in healthy control subjects, is significantly impaired in patients with ASPD and even more so in patients with psychopathy.

E. Patients with ASPD and patients with psychopathy have similar findings on frontal imaging studies.

CHAPTER 6

Prevalence, Sociodemographics, and Functional Impairment

6.1   In the general population, what is the approximate prevalence for any personality disorder (PD)?

   A. <1%.
   B. Between 1% and 2%.
   C. Between 3% and 5%.
   D. Between 10% and 15%.
   E. Between 20% and 25%.

6.2   Which PD occurs most frequently in the general population?

   A. Antisocial PD.
   B. Borderline PD (BPD).
   C. Dependent PD.
   D. Narcissistic PD.
   E. Obsessive-compulsive PD.

6.3   How do point prevalence rates of PDs change over a lifetime?

   A. Rates increase as the population ages.
   B. Rates decrease as the population ages.
   C. Rates are mostly constant as the population ages.
   D. Rates vary unpredictably as the population ages.
   E. Rates increase until age 50 and then decrease.

6.4   Which PD is much more prevalent in the clinical population than in the general population?

A. BPD.
B. Obsessive-compulsive PD.
C. Paranoid PD.
D. Passive-aggressive PD.
E. Schizoid PD.

6.5   What developmental trend is observed in Cluster B PDs compared with Cluster A PDs?

A. Persons with Cluster B PDs tend to be younger.
B. Persons with Cluster B PDs tend to be older.
C. Persons with Cluster B PDs tend to be middle-aged.
D. Persons with Cluster B PDs are just as likely to be any age.
E. Persons with Cluster A and B PDs tend to be similar ages.

6.6   Although many PDs are related to lower education, which PD goes against this trend and seems to be correlated with higher education?

A. Histrionic PD.
B. Narcissistic PD.
C. Obsessive-compulsive PD.
D. Paranoid PD.
E. Schizoid PD.

6.7   What is the relationship between quality of life and number of criteria fulfilled for any specific PD?

A. Quality of life decreases with increasing number of criteria fulfilled in a linear relationship.
B. Quality of life is associated with number of criteria fulfilled only to a limited extent.
C. Quality of life is equally affected beyond a certain number of fulfilled criteria.
D. Quality of life and number of criteria show a relationship in only certain PDs.
E. Quality of life is affected only after reaching a certain threshold of criteria fulfilled.

6.8   Which PD is associated with the highest levels of dysfunction and poorest quality of life?

A. Avoidant PD.
B. BPD.
C. Dependent PD.
D. Histrionic PD.
E. Obsessive-compulsive PD.

6.9   Which of the following individuals is most likely to have a diagnosis of a PD?

   A. A 25-year-old male medical student living with his wife in the suburbs.
   B. A 26-year-old separated female with an associate's degree living in a rural area.
   C. A 27-year-old female with a GED living with her partner on the outskirts of a city.
   D. A 28-year-old divorced man without a high school degree living alone in a city.
   E. A 29-year-old single woman working as an attorney in a metropolitan area.

6.10   Which of the following PDs is more common in women?

   A. Antisocial PD.
   B. BPD.
   C. Dependent PD.
   D. Schizoid PD.
   E. Schizotypal PD.

Manifestations, Assessment, and Differential Diagnosis

7.1 DSM-5 Section III provides diagnostic criteria for which of the following personality disorders (PDs)?

    A. Dependent.
    B. Histrionic.
    C. Paranoid.
    D. Schizoid.
    E. Schizotypal.

7.2 Criterion A of the general criteria for the diagnosis of PD in the alternative DSM-5 model of PD requires moderate or greater impairment in which of the following areas of personality functioning?

    A. Conscientiousness.
    B. Emotional stability.
    C. Extraversion.
    D. Lucidity.
    E. Self/interpersonal relatedness.

7.3 Which one of the following is one of the five broad pathological personality trait domains in DSM-5 Section III?

    A. Detachment.
    B. Submissiveness.
    C. Impulsivity.
    D. Manipulativeness.
    E. Eccentricity.

7.4   In DSM-5 Section III, alternative diagnostic model of PDs, the Level of Personality Functioning Scale (LPFS) assesses which of the following areas of personality and adaptive functioning?

    A. Agreeableness.
    B. Conscientiousness.
    C. Empathy.
    D. Extroversion.
    E. Openness.

7.5   Which of the following PDs is least likely to have impairment in the domains of social, work, and leisure?

    A. Avoidant.
    B. Borderline.
    C. Obsessive-compulsive.
    D. Schizotypal.

7.6   Agreement between the patient and an informant about personality traits and interpersonal problems is highest for which of the following PDs?

    A. Avoidant.
    B. Borderline.
    C. Dependent.
    D. Narcissistic.
    E. Paranoid.

7.7   Which is the only PD that cannot be diagnosed before age 18 years?

    A. Antisocial.
    B. Avoidant.
    C. Borderline.
    D. Dependent.
    E. Schizotypal.

7.8   Which PD may become more pronounced with age?

    A. Antisocial.
    B. Avoidant.
    C. Paranoid.
    D. Dependent.
    E. Schizotypal.

7.9 The externalizing "meta-cluster" of disorders is characterized primarily by which of the following personality traits?

A. Detachment.
B. Disinhibition.
C. Extraversion.
D. Negative affectivity.
E. Psychoticism.

7.10 As part of the assessment in the outpatient psychiatric clinic, a patient is administered the Personality Inventory for DSM-5 (PID-5). The patient scores high on the PID-5 on traits of negative affectivity, antagonism, and disinhibition. On the basis of these findings, which of the PDs is the most likely diagnosis for this patient?

A. Antisocial.
B. Avoidant.
C. Borderline.
D. Narcissistic.
E. Schizotypal.

CHAPTER 8

Course and Outcome

8.1 Which of the following is a key concept of personality disorders (PDs) in both the DSM-5 and the ICD-10?

A. Classification of categories.
B. Definitions of traits.
C. Criteria for diagnosis.
D. Stability over time.
E. Impact on function.

8.2 According to Carpenter and Gunderson, the impairment in functioning observed for borderline PD (BPD) over a 5-year period was comparable to the impairment of functioning in patients with which of the following disorders?

A. Major depression.
B. Bipolar disorder.
C. Panic disorder.
D. Social phobia.
E. Schizophrenia.

8.3 What was the intent in DSM-III to place the PDs on a separate axis (Axis II) of the multiaxial system?

A. Assess for presence of disorders often overlooked in the presence of an Axis I disorder.
B. Diagnostic construct of PD did not evolve over time.
C. Recognize the instability of both Axis I and Axis II PDs.
D. Encourage clinicians to focus on a specific disorder.
E. Recognize the pattern of instability of personality traits.

8.4 The placement of PDs on a separate axis facilitated which of the following research issues?

A. Increased research focus on Axis I disorders.
B. Development and utilization of structured and standardized clinical interviewing.

C. Recognition of the effect of Axis I disorders on PDs.

D. Increased accuracy of diagnosis of the different PDs.

E. Increased accuracy of diagnosis of Axis I disorders.

8.5 Research regarding the long-term course of PDs involves the repeated-measures approach (test-retest), which may address the problem of "regression to the mean." What is an untoward effect on the reliability of study data caused by this methodology?

A. Participants systematically report or endorse fewer problems on repeat interview by reporting fewer symptoms.

B. Participants prefer to remain in one study for an extended duration.

C. Participants will have a tendency to underreport symptoms at baseline.

D. Participants tend to report more symptoms on repeat interview to increase interview times.

E. Participants become more consistent on repeat interview over an extended period of time.

8.6 If diagnosed during adolescence, which of the following diagnoses predicts substantially elevated risk for antisocial behavior during adulthood?

A. Attention-deficit/hyperactivity disorder.

B. Bipolar disorder.

C. Conduct disorder.

D. Obsessive-compulsive disorder.

E. Social phobia.

8.7 Why is determining early onset of PDs in adolescence difficult?

A. Consistency of personality traits decreases with age.

B. Consistency of personality traits is highest during adolescence.

C. Adolescents are unreliable in their self-report to the structured interviews.

D. Adolescence is a period of profound changes and flux in personality and identity.

E. The effect of peer pressure during adolescence confounds the presentation of personality traits.

8.8 The temperamental feature of being withdrawn in childhood is noted to be a precursor of which of the following PDs in adulthood?

A. Avoidant.

B. Borderline.

C. Dependent.

D. Paranoid.

E. Schizotypal.

8.9 Which of the following PD clusters tends to show significant improvement with age?

A. Cluster A.
B. Cluster B.
C. Cluster C.

8.10 Which of the following PDs is associated with a significantly longer duration of time to achieve remission (defined as good social and vocational functioning in addition to minimal PD symptoms) than all other PDs?

A. Avoidant.
B. Histrionic.
C. Borderline.
D. Paranoid.
E. Schizoid.

8.11 What did the 10 years of prospective yearly multimethod follow-up in the Collaborative Longitudinal Personality Disorders Study (CLPS) demonstrate about the course of BPD?

A. High rates of diagnostic remission and low rates of relapse (return to diagnostic threshold), but severe and enduring social functioning impairment.
B. Low rates of diagnostic remission and low rates of relapse (return to diagnostic threshold), but severe and enduring social functioning impairment.
C. High rates of diagnostic remission and high rates of relapse (return to diagnostic threshold), but severe and enduring social functioning impairment.
D. Low rates of diagnostic remission and high rates of relapse (return to diagnostic threshold), but severe and enduring social functioning impairment.
E. High rates of diagnostic remission, low rates of relapse (return to diagnostic threshold), and decreased social functioning impairment.

CHAPTER 9

Therapeutic Alliance

9.1   In research on the treatment of personality disorders (PDs), which of the following is the most robust predictor of treatment outcome?

A. Therapeutic alliance.
B. Duration of therapy.
C. Therapeutic modality.
D. Socioeconomic factors.
E. Self-harm history.

9.2   The concept of therapeutic alliance is attributed originally to which of the following people?

A. Gerald Adler.
B. Heinz Kohut.
C. Otto Kernberg.
D. Sigmund Freud.
E. Donald Winnicott.

9.3   A patient who has had a good therapeutic alliance with his psychiatrist for a year suddenly appears dissatisfied with the treatment during a session. He calls later and leaves a message wanting to discontinue therapy. Which of the following is the recommended therapist response?

A. Transfer the patient to the care of another psychiatrist.
B. Suggest the patient return to share his concerns.
C. Refer the patient to the state medical board complaints office.
D. Contact a lawyer for medicolegal advice.
E. Discuss the case with another psychiatrist to review therapist counter-transference.

9.4   Which of the following is a characteristic clinical challenge when treating a patient with a Cluster A (paranoid/schizoid/schizotypal) PD?

A. Establishing a working alliance with the patient.
B. Unstable emotional and cognitive states of the patient.
C. Patient sensitivity to treatment recommendations as criticism.
D. Patient's need for control of the treatment process.
E. Addressing patient's demandingness.

9.5   A patient who starts therapy with a new psychiatrist is very complimentary at the first appointment. By the third appointment, the patient voices numerous verbal criticisms and expresses anger with the clinical treatment. There are no inappropriate threats or concerns to the psychiatrist's safety, and the patient makes another appointment. Which of the following is the most helpful response the psychiatrist could employ for this patient?

A. Terminate therapy and discharge the patient.
B. Contact a malpractice lawyer for advice.
C. Interpret the reason for the anger.
D. Tolerate the expression of anger.
E. Identify and explain the development of transference.

9.6   Which of the following is the appropriate therapeutic stance in the early stages of treatment with a patient who has narcissistic PD?

A. Tolerate the patient's grandiosity.
B. Agree with the patient's sense of self-importance.
C. Firmly establish and demonstrate therapist control.
D. Use numerous early interpretations.
E. Ask for proof of grandiose claims.

9.7   With respect to the his or her therapeutic alliance, which of the following is characteristic of a person with Cluster C PDs during treatment?

A. Feels guilt and takes blame for situations with the therapist.
B. Develops a quick and deep alliance with the therapist.
C. Frequently alternates between idealizing and devaluing the therapist.
D. Has difficulty trusting the therapist.
E. Exploits and uses the therapist to gratify personal needs.

9.8   When providing therapy to a person with borderline PD (BPD), which of the following approaches carries the greatest risk of rupturing the therapeutic alliance?

A. Supportive psychotherapy.
B. Cognitive-behavioral therapy.
C. Psychoeducation.
D. Medication management.
E. Transference interpretations.

9.9 What is the recommended physician stance when prescribing medication to patients with PDs?

A. Directive expert.
B. Collaborative participant.
C. Passive responder.
D. Authoritarian leader.
E. Interpretive reflector.

9.10 During the inpatient hospitalization of a patient with BPD, a treatment team encounters escalating conflict with each other about the treatment. Which of the following is the recommended action?

A. Transfer the patient to a different unit.
B. Change the attending psychiatrist.
C. Have team members independently assess the patient and contribute opinions.
D. Request a second opinion to decide on treatment.
E. Hold a team meeting to communicate and have a common united approach.

CHAPTER 10

Psychodynamic Psychotherapies and Psychoanalysis

10.1 Which of the following best describes the criteria for a diagnosis of borderline personality organization?

A. The patient's personality organization is characterized by primitive defense mechanisms, identity diffusion, and generally intact but unstable reality testing.
B. The patient's personality is characterized by primitive defense mechanisms, identity diffusion, and loss of reality testing.
C. The patient's personality organization is characterized by primitive defense mechanisms, an overly consolidated identity, and generally intact but unstable reality testing.
D. The patient's personality organization is characterized by primitive defense mechanisms, identity diffusion, and the patient meets DSM criteria for borderline personality disorder (BPD).
E. The patient's personality organization is characterized by primitive defense mechanisms and the patient meets criteria for any of the personality disorders (PDs) described in the DSM.

10.2 Which of the following psychological mechanisms are most central to a psychoanalytic understanding of severe PDs?

A. Repression and reaction formation.
B. Splitting and projective identification.
C. Humor and sublimation.
D. A neurotic level of personality organization.
E. Significant absence of reality testing.

10.3 Which of the following is true of specific psychoanalytic schools of thought as they relate to PDs?

A. In conceptualizing PDs, self psychology places special emphasis on the importance of psychological conflicts.
B. In conceptualizing PDs, ego psychology places more emphasis than other schools on the role of deficient child rearing in giving rise to PDs.
C. In conceptualizing PDs, object relations theory focuses on the importance of mental representations of self and others.
D. In conceptualizing PDs, the relational and interpersonal schools of psychoanalysis understand pathological traits in terms of the interpersonal expression of inner aggressive drives.
E. In conceptualizing personality pathology, mentalization-based therapy (MBT) focuses on how inherited difficulties with mentalization, rather than childhood trauma, give rise to pathological character traits.

10.4 Which of the following is true regarding the appropriateness of psychoanalytic treatment for patients with PDs?

A. Psychoanalysis is not an effective treatment for PDs, and patients should be referred for treatment with other modalities.
B. Psychoanalysis is effective for patients with less severe PDs and requires no modifications for patients with more severe PDs.
C. Psychoanalysis may be an effective treatment for some patients without PDs but is rarely useful for patients with PDs.
D. Psychoanalysis has become a viable alternative for working with severe PDs as appropriate technical modifications have been developed and tested.
E. Psychoanalysis should never be a first-line treatment for any patients with a PD.

10.5 Which of the following modalities of psychotherapy for PDs involves a combination of group sessions and individual sessions; focuses on the patient's capacity to reflect on and appreciate intentions, feelings, and motivations in self and others; and, in later stages of treatment, works toward achieving such reflective functioning in the patient-therapist interaction?

A. Transference-focused psychotherapy (TFP).
B. Supportive-expressive therapy.
C. Dialectical behavioral therapy (DBT).
D. Psychoanalysis.
E. MBT.

10.6 According to the theory underlying MBT, which of the following early life conditions are related to later failures in mentalization?

A. Attunement difficulties between the infant and the caretaker impede a secure sense of attachment.
B. The child has a punitive superego.
C. The infant fails to integrate good and bad experiences of self and others.
D. Caregivers are not available to affirm, and to be idealized by, the child, who therefore does not develop a cohesive sense of self.
E. The child has a weak ego and uses primitive defenses.

10.7 Which of the following best describes the relative roles of supportive techniques and expressive techniques in the major psychodynamic approaches to treating PDs?

A. All approaches to the psychodynamic treatment of PDs prioritize expressive techniques over supportive techniques.
B. Some approaches to the psychodynamic treatment of PDs emphasize expressive techniques over supportive techniques, some emphasize supportive techniques over expressive techniques, and some emphasize a mix of supportive and expressive techniques.
C. All approaches to the psychodynamic treatment of PDs prioritize supportive techniques over expressive techniques.
D. All approaches to the psychodynamic treatment of PDs emphasize a mix of supportive and expressive techniques.
E. The distinction between supportive techniques and expressive techniques is less relevant to the psychodynamic treatment of patients with PDs than it is to the psychodynamic treatment of patients without PDs.

10.8 Which of the following modalities of psychodynamic psychotherapy for PDs involves twice-weekly meetings; a focus on the treatment contract prior to beginning treatment; and an emphasis on clarification, confrontation, and early interpretation of representations of self and others as they emerge in the transference?

A. MBT.
B. Supportive-expressive therapy.
C. TFP.
D. Psychoanalysis.
E. Supportive psychotherapy.

10.9 Which of the following is true of the evidence basis for psychodynamic treatment of PDs?

A. Across diagnoses, evidence supporting the use of cognitive-behavioral therapy (CBT) far outweighs evidence supporting the use of psychodynamic psychotherapy.
B. There is little empirical evidence that psychodynamic psychotherapy is useful in the treatment of PDs.
C. Transference interpretations, which are central to psychoanalytic or psychodynamic psychotherapy, have been shown to be most effective with psychologically minded patients and least effective with patients who are not psychologically minded.
D. Several modalities of psychodynamic psychotherapy have been demonstrated to be effective in the treatment of PDs.
E. TFP has been found to be less effective than either DBT or supportive psychotherapy when treating patients with PDs who are not psychologically minded.

10.10 The related concepts of object relations dyads and internal working models are derived from which of the theoretical schools listed below?

A. Object relations theory and attachment theory.
B. Self psychology and attachment theory.
C. Object relations theory and ego psychology.
D. Libido theory and ego psychology.
E. Attachment theory and ego psychology.

CHAPTER 11

Cognitive-Behavioral Therapy I: Basics and Principles

11.1 Which of the following represents a central therapeutic goal of contemporary cognitive-behavioral treatment for personality disorders (PDs)?

   A. The therapist should seek to change the patient's basic assumptions and cognitions.
   B. The therapist should assist the patient in linking mood fluctuations to interpersonal situations.
   C. The therapist should encourage patients to practice goal-oriented behavior in the face of dysfunctional cognitions.
   D. The therapist should guide the patient toward uncovering the role of unconscious conflict in maintaining maladaptive behaviors.
   E. The therapist should guide the patient away from any psychopharmacologic treatments.

11.2 Empirically validated treatment recommendations currently exist for which of the following PDs?

   A. Narcissistic.
   B. Obsessive-compulsive.
   C. Histrionic.
   D. Avoidant.
   E. Schizoid.

11.3 Which of the following factors is *most* relevant to consider when planning cognitive-behavioral treatment for a patient with a PD?

   A. External social variables.
   B. Family history of suicide.
   C. Prior medication trials.
   D. Prior psychiatric admissions.
   E. Insurance and financial resources.

11.4   A 27-year-old woman with BPD is in weekly psychotherapy. Her therapist goes on vacation for 2 weeks, during which time the patient experiences a recurrence of self-injurious behavior. How would a cognitive-behavioral therapist describe this patient's behavior?

   A. Goal-related behavior.
   B. Transference reaction.
   C. Treatment-interfering behavior.
   D. Acting-out behavior.
   E. Crisis-generating behavior.

11.5   After several months of CBT, a 35-year-old man with avoidant PD decides to attend a social gathering. Fifteen minutes into the party he leaves because he thinks the other guests find him awkward and inadequate. How would a cognitive-behavioral therapist describe this phenomenon?

   A. Defense against anticipated rejection.
   B. Dysfunctional misinterpretation.
   C. Anxiety over dependency needs.
   D. Interpersonal deficits.
   E. Avoidant attachment style.

11.6   Which of the following is a true statement about psychoeducation in the cognitive-behavioral treatment of patients with PDs?

   A. Patients should not be told their diagnosis because it will increase risk of suicide.
   B. Patients have a right to be told their diagnosis, and concealing this information is an ethical violation.
   C. Informing patients with PDs about their diagnosis is a straightforward aspect of psychoeducation that is rarely debated.
   D. Only patients with Cluster C PDs should be informed of their diagnosis.
   E. For selected PDs, the benefits of openly communicating the diagnosis mostly outweigh the disadvantages.

11.7   Which of the following is true of therapy contracts in cognitive-behavioral treatment of patients with PDs?

   A. Therapy contracts should include discussion of expected duration and frequency of treatment.
   B. Discussion of suicidal crises and behavior is not typically addressed in cognitive-behavioral treatment contracts.
   C. Patients with PDs should not be told how to reach the therapist in case of emergency because they are likely to abuse this privilege.
   D. Therapy contracts for patients with PDs are no different than those for patients with other psychiatric diagnoses.
   E. Patients with PDs should not be informed of the therapist's training and supervision.

11.8 A 52-year-old man with narcissistic PD has been in regular CBT for 1 month and has developed a good therapeutic alliance. When his therapist is 10 minutes late for a session, the patient angrily says, "What a fool I am for thinking you were better than the rest of the world out there…turns out you are no different. …You are incompetent and of no use to me." Which of the following is the correct response for the therapist to make to the patient?

   A. The therapist stays silent and expressionless, waiting to see what the patient will say next.
   B. "You are being extremely rude. This behavior is unacceptable and I will be unable to continue the session if you cannot calm down."
   C. "I am sorry that I was late. I see that you are angry and with good reason. Nevertheless, your behavior right now is making me feel rather helpless. Is that your intention?"
   D. "I am sorry that I was late. Tell me what it felt like to be kept waiting."
   E. "You are clearly feeling hurt and disappointed, and I think you are taking that out on me to punish me and make me feel what you are feeling. This is what you do with the rest of the world, and it is why you are so alone and miserable."

11.9 Which of the following is an exercise that a patient in CBT may practice in order to help identify dysfunctional information processing?

   A. Mindfulness meditation.
   B. Analysis of transference.
   C. Interpersonal inventory.
   D. Behavioral or chain analysis.
   E. Dream analysis.

11.10 A 47-year-old woman with paranoid PD is in weekly CBT. She tells her therapist that her coworker has been more aloof lately and is "probably getting cozy with the boss to try to edge me out and make me look bad." Which of the following would be a correct CBT response?

   A. "You sound very angry at your coworker; I think you are projecting your hostility."
   B. "Could there be another possible explanation for your coworker's recent behavior?"
   C. "You are using the cognitive distortion of 'mind reading.' Let's try to change that."
   D. "It sounds like you feel threatened by your coworker. What comes to mind about that?"
   E. "You are responding to your coworker the same way you did to your sister growing up when you felt excluded and inferior."

CHAPTER 12

Cognitive-Behavioral Therapy II: Specific Strategies for Personality Disorders

12.1 What does the cognitive-behavioral therapy (CBT) technique of cognitive restructuring emphasize in the treatment of patients with personality disorders (PDs)?

A. How the thought process functions within the person's life.
B. The content of the negative thoughts.
C. Preventing nonsuicidal self-injury (NSSI).
D. Relationship to managing negative emotions.
E. Irrational thoughts without consideration to context.

12.2 In using CBT with patients with PDs, what is the most important feature of setting treatment goals?

A. Flexibility.
B. Collaboration.
C. Noncritical statements.
D. Focusing on interpersonal relationships.
E. Addressing nonsuicidal self-injurious behavior.

12.3 A 25-year-old female patient presents with symptoms consistent with borderline PD (BPD). She reports that her greatest concern, and reason for seeking treatment, is unstable relationships with men, friends, and family. Her father has always been verbally abusive and her mother has been emotionally unavailable because of severe depression. The patient experiences her early and current home environment as critical and invalidating. She has developed a view of herself as worthless and a view of others as rejecting. When she perceives rejection, she is prone to intense anger, acting impulsively or engaging in nonsuicidal self-injurious behavior. On the basis of the research and her beliefs about self and others, which type of CBT should be considered and will likely be most effective?

A. Acceptance and commitment therapy.
B. Dialectical behavior therapy (DBT).
C. Schema-focused therapy (SFT).
D. Mindfulness-based treatment.
E. Cognitive-analytic therapy.

12.4   For which PD has research shown modest effects for CBT but not demonstrated superiority over treatment as usual (TAU)?

A. Dependent PD.
B. Schizotypal PD.
C. BPD.
D. Histrionic PD.
E. Antisocial PD.

12.5   What is a newer form of CBT that is currently being explored and adapted to treatment of PDs?

A. DBT.
B. Psychodynamic therapy.
C. Acceptance and commitment therapy.
D. Interpersonal therapy.
E. SFT.

12.6   Therapist effects were found to be significant in the Borderline Personality Disorder Study of Cognitive Therapy, a well-designed randomized clinical trial to test efficacy of CBT (Davidson et al. 2006). With which of the following provided by the therapists did patients have two to three times greater improvement in suicide-related outcomes?

A. Emergency services and medication management.
B. Cognitive techniques to modify core beliefs and schemas.
C. Behavioral strategies to promote adaptive functioning.
D. Higher quantity and more competent delivery of CBT.
E. Exposure to situations that triggered emotional distress.

12.7   What is a major difference between DBT and traditional CBT?

A. Maladaptive behaviors are viewed with acceptance and validation.
B. Historical context is considered in the development of negative cognitions.
C. Solid empirical evidence exists to support effectiveness.
D. NSSI is monitored and addressed.
E. Skills training is emphasized.

12.8   What did the results of randomized clinical trials consistently show for group-based cognitive-behavioral treatments for PDs?

   A. Significant reduction of NSSI behavior.
   B. Superiority over TAU.
   C. No difference as compared with TAU.
   D. Greater effectiveness as compared with psychodynamic therapy.
   E. Equally as effective as individual CBT.

12.9   Which of the models used in DSM-5 for PDs best matches with a CBT treatment approach?

   A. Dimensional model.
   B. Categorical model.
   C. Cluster trait model.
   D. Quantitative hierarchical model.
   E. Hybrid Axis I and II model.

12.10   Which of the following describes the current American Psychiatric Association (APA) treatment guideline for patients with BPD?

   A. Pharmacotherapy only.
   B. Primary treatment of pharmacotherapy with adjunctive psychotherapy.
   C. Primary treatment of CBT.
   D. Primary treatment of psychotherapy with adjunctive, symptom-targeted pharmacotherapy.
   E. Pharmacotherapy with psychotherapy for anxiety, depressive, or substance abuse disorders as indicated.

CHAPTER 13

Group, Family, and Couples Therapies

13.1 What feature of personality disorders (PDs) makes group therapy, with its frequent verbal and nonverbal exchanges with others, particularly effective?

    A. Patients are frequently oblivious to their interpersonal maladaptive behaviors.
    B. Patients may have intrapersonal difficulties.
    C. Patients may be prone to emotional outbursts.
    D. Patients with self-injurious behaviors can benefit from expressing threats of harmful behavior.
    E. Aggressive or threatening behaviors are mitigated in the group setting.

13.2 How do patients with PDs more typically reveal their pathology, which may facilitate group treatment?

    A. Describing in words.
    B. Demonstrating in action.
    C. Dealing with internally.
    D. Defending against subconsciously.
    E. Deliberating carefully.

13.3 Which PDs are associated with the role of therapist helper in the group therapy setting?

    A. Antisocial PD and narcissistic PD.
    B. Dependent PD and histrionic PD.
    C. Paranoid PD and avoidant PD.
    D. Obsessive-compulsive PD and borderline PD (BPD).
    E. Schizoid PD and schizotypal PD.

13.4 What is the role of the therapist when a patient is identified as a difficult group member?

A. Ask the patient to leave the group.
B. Discern whether the individual may be serving a defensive function for the group.
C. Ask the patient during the group why he or she is being difficult so that the group can contribute to the discussion.
D. Avoid bringing attention to the problem so that the patient's feelings are not hurt.
E. Invite the patient to join an alternative group to see if the problems continue.

13.5 What PD was the Systems Training for Emotional Predictability and Problem Solving (STEPPS) group therapy initially designed to target?

A. Narcissistic PD.
B. Histrionic PD.
C. Dependent PD.
D. Avoidant PD.
E. BPD.

13.6 What is the definition in terms of duration for long-term outpatient group therapy?

A. 12 weeks.
B. 6 months.
C. 1 year.
D. 2 years.
E. 3 years.

13.7 In what way has dialectical behavioral therapy (DBT) been shown to be superior with respect to the following to treatment as usual?

A. Suicidal and self-injurious behaviors.
B. Distress.
C. Interpersonal problems.
D. Regulation of emotion.
E. Mindfulness.

13.8 Which psychoanalytically oriented day treatment program combines group and individual therapy and is unique in the long follow-up period studied?

A. DBT.
B. Mentalization-based therapy.
C. Cognitive-behavioral therapy (CBT).
D. STEPPS.
E. Interpersonal psychotherapy.

13.9   In which of the following situations might family therapy for treatment of a PD
        be contraindicated?

        A. Family consists of more than five individuals.
        B. Family includes more than one member with a PD.
        C. Family includes a member who feels overwhelming embarrassment when dis-
           cussing personal issues in front of family.
        D. Family includes a member who is in individual therapy.
        E. Family has multiple interpersonal difficulties.

13.10   What is the effect of a positive romantic relationship on BPD?

        A. No effect.
        B. Healing effect.
        C. Increased impulsivity.
        D. Decreased functioning.
        E. Increased regression.

13.11   In DBT adapted for couples, dialectics include which of the following?

        A. Intimacy versus autonomy.
        B. Autonomy versus shame and doubt.
        C. Intimacy versus isolation.
        D. Trust versus mistrust.
        E. Initiative versus guilt.

CHAPTER 14

Psychoeducation

14.1   Which of the following statements comparing psychoeducation and psychother-
        apy is true?

   A. As with psychotherapy, the methods and procedures of psychoeducation are
      both educational and therapeutic.
   B. Psychotherapy has been shown to reduce recurrence, which is not true for psy-
      choeducation.
   C. Unlike psychotherapy, individuals in recovery or family members frequently
      deliver psychoeducation.
   D. In contrast with psychotherapy, psychoeducation has yet to establish efficacy
      beyond Axis I disorders.
   E. Psychoeducation, unlike psychotherapy, is evidence-based.

14.2   Which focus of psychoeducation is thought to be most relevant to short-term and
        long-term patient outcomes?

   A. Current family functioning factors.
   B. Knowledge base alone.
   C. Specific etiologic pathways for personality disorder (PD).
   D. Existing treatment options, including medications and therapy.
   E. Developmental history of the patient.

14.3   Which core component is least consistently found in psychoeducational pro-
        grams?

   A. Education.
   B. Problem solving.
   C. Social support.
   D. Skills training.
   E. Bibliotherapy.

14.4 Which statement is most accurate regarding psychoeducation for PDs?

A. Psychoeducation programs have been developed widely for several of the PDs.
B. Psychoeducation programs for antisocial PD have demonstrated a reduction in violence recidivism.
C. There are some data to suggest psychoeducation is contraindicated for Cluster B disorders.
D. Several studies have shown positive outcomes using psychoeducation in combination with other interventions in avoidant PD.
E. A number of patient and family psychoeducation programs have been developed for Cluster A diagnoses because programs for related Axis I disorders have been successful.

14.5 In discussion with a patient, it becomes clear her sister has BPD. Which of the following is the best psychoeducational approach to informing the patient about her sister?

A. Suggest that she search the Internet for information on BPD.
B. Describe for her the homogeneous nature of the disorder.
C. Explain how stability across time distinguishes PD from other psychiatric disorders.
D. Note that for BPD we do not yet know what is inherited, what is learned, or how these factors interact.
E. Warn the patient that her sister may have suffered a significant trauma, because trauma is a necessary and sufficient cause of BPD.

14.6 A colleague asks your thoughts on how to advise her new patient with BPD about treatment options. A psychoeducational approach to informing the patient about treatment should include which of the following?

A. Advise that in terms of evidence-based treatments, mentalization-based therapy has the most supporting studies, with dozens of controlled and uncontrolled trials.
B. Reassure the patient that there are an increasing variety of treatments for BPD and that the vast majority of BPD patients have access to them.
C. Note that it is unreasonable for the patient and her family to have a timetable in mind for recovery.
D. Suggest that if there are no BPD-specific treatments available to the patient, it is more prudent to forgo treatment and instead seek peer support.
E. Inform the patient that there is no medication that is consistently or dramatically helpful in the treatment of BPD.

14.7 Which statement most accurately describes the joining phase of Gunderson's multifamily groups for BPD?

A. Relatives from one family join a multifamily group to create an alliance and connection with other families.
B. General information about BPD is provided, but information about family members' history is not elicited.
C. During this phase, acknowledgement of family members' anger and angst is avoided because it undermines the alliance with the patient.
D. The joining phase offers participants the experience of hearing from other families in similar situations.
E. Participants nearing completion of this phase are asked to commit, in general, to a 4-month period for the remainder of this phase of treatment.

14.8 Which of the following statements does *not* describe DBT-oriented family skills training (DBT-FST)?

A. It offers a forum to put skill acquisition and generalization practice into the family environment.
B. It was developed specifically for family participants, and patients do not attend the sessions.
C. It attempts to educate family participants about BPD.
D. It works to teach a new language of communication based on DBT skills.
E. It promotes an attitude that is nonjudgmental, which is particularly useful for high-stress participant families.

14.9 In which psychoeducation program does the patient assume the role of co-teacher to inform and educate those people important to him or her?

A. Gunderson's multifamily groups.
B. Systems Training for Emotional Predictability and Problem Solving (STEPPS).
C. Family Connections.
D. DBT- FST.
E. Peer specialist program.

14.10 A 24-year-old woman was recently diagnosed with BPD. Her parents are distressed because the patient refuses to engage in any treatment. The patient's parents feel confused and isolated. What program might be appropriate for the parents?

A. Gunderson's multifamily groups.
B. STEPPS.
C. Family Connections.
D. DBT- FST.
E. Peer specialist program.

CHAPTER 15

Somatic Treatments

15.1   Which of the following medications has been shown to worsen impulsivity and behavioral dyscontrol in individuals with borderline personality disorder (BPD)?

A. Alprazolam.
B. Fluoxetine.
C. Haloperidol.
D. Lamotrigine.
E. Lithium.

15.2   Which of the following medications has been shown to reduce psychoticism in patients with schizotypal PD?

A. Aripiprazole.
B. Clozapine.
C. Quetiapine.
D. Risperidone.
E. Ziprasidone.

15.3   Which of the following antidepressants has been associated with worsening of symptoms of BPD?

A. Amitriptyline.
B. Fluoxetine.
C. Phenelzine.
D. Selegiline.
E. Venlafaxine.

15.4   Which of the following medications has been shown to be helpful in patients with BPD who do not respond to selective serotonin reuptake inhibitors (SSRIs)?

A. Clonazepam.
B. Haloperidol.
C. Lithium.
D. Omega-3 fatty acids.
E. Venlafaxine.

15.5 Which of the following symptom domains in BPD were improved during treatment with omega-3 fatty acids?

A. Aggression.
B. Anxiety.
C. Impulsivity.
D. Mood lability.
E. Suicidality.

15.6 What is the best recommendation for appropriate use of medications in the treatment of BPD?

A. Acute use of medications targeted to specific symptom domains.
B. Acute use of medications to prepare the patient to enter psychotherapy.
C. Avoidance of medications during psychotherapy.
D. Chronic use of medications in patients unable to engage in psychotherapy.
E. Chronic use of medications to reduce overall BPD severity.

15.7 On the basis of the results of a large meta-analysis of controlled trials, psychopharmacologic medications have the largest effect size for treatment of which of the following symptom domains in BPD?

A. Anxiety.
B. Cognitive-perceptual disturbances.
C. Depressed mood.
D. Emptiness.
E. Impulsive-behavioral dyscontrol.

15.8 Which of the following PDs has the strongest evidence base to support the use of psychopharmacologic treatment?

A. Avoidant PD.
B. BPD.
C. Obsessive-compulsive PD.
D. Schizoid PD.
E. Schizotypal PD.

15.9 A 26-year-old patient presents with complaints of mood swings in the context of a recent breakup. She has recently moved and is seeking a new psychiatrist. She states that she has always had problems keeping a relationship for more than a couple of months, noting that the relationship seems "perfect" at first but then suddenly and inexplicably seems to end. She experiences mood swings, intense anger, irritability, and anxiety. She states that she "hates" herself and notes that everyone important in her life has always let her down. She also has a history of making superficial lacerations to her wrists, but she firmly denies any current suicidal thoughts or plans. She is currently taking alprazolam 0.5 mg three times daily, fluoxetine 40 mg daily, and risperidone 2 mg nightly. In addition to active engagement in psychotherapy, which of the following is the most appropriate next step in her treatment?

A. Add valproate.
B. Change fluoxetine to venlafaxine.
C. Increase fluoxetine.
D. Increase risperidone.
E. Taper and discontinue alprazolam.

CHAPTER 16
Collaborative Treatment

16.1   What is the best definition of collaborative treatment?

    A. A method of delivering cognitive-behavioral therapy (CBT).
    B. A treatment relationship that occurs when two or more treatment modalities are provided by more than one mental health or medical professional.
    C. A system of care that is only delivered in a particular setting.
    D. A treatment that used to be delivered in the primary care setting but has not persisted.

16.2   *Split treatment* may be viewed as one form of collaborative treatment. How is split treatment different from collaborative care?

    A. There is often a lack of communication or agreement between the providers.
    B. The bills for care of the patient are split.
    C. There is a split in the unconscious and conscious realm of care.
    D. The patient realizes that he or she must split his or her time between the hospital and outpatient services.

16.3   What is a problem that may occur in split treatment of patients with PDs?

    A. Most patients with schizoid traits may ask for increased doses of antidepressants.
    B. There are fewer prescriptions for mood stabilizers.
    C. Patients with Cluster C traits may become increasingly obsessional.
    D. Patients with Cluster B traits tend to split even without a split treatment relationship.

16.4   Why is it important to employ collaborative treatment for patients with PDs?

    A. Efficacy studies within this patient population demonstrate superiority of multiple care providers over just one provider.
    B. Many patients with PDs often do not respond as well to medications as would patients with other primary diagnoses and thus may need other treatment modalities.
    C. Families generally ask for many clinicians to care for their loved one.
    D. Strong comparison data show that pharmacotherapy and psychotherapy are only useful in a minority subset of patients with PDs.

16.5   Patients are increasingly receiving most psychotropic medication prescriptions from which of the following professionals?

A. Cardiologists.

B. Primary care physicians.

C. Psychiatrists.

D. Social workers.

16.6   A managed care company would be most likely to agree with which of the following statements about patients with PDs?

A. They use much less than their share of psychiatric treatment.

B. They use just enough of their share of psychiatric treatment.

C. They should be encouraged to take full advantage of their psychiatric benefit.

D. They use too much or at least more than their share of treatment benefits.

16.7   Patients with PDs often have mixtures of symptoms and problems, some of which
arise from psychosocial issues and others from baseline anxiety, emotional lability, and impulsivity. Which is most likely to occur in the split treatment of a patient
with a PD?

A. The psychotherapist may believe that most of the problems arise from psychosocial issues and may be dismissive of the psychopharmacological treatment.

B. The psychopharmacologist may feel that the difficulties are all due to "trait expression" and not prescribe antidepressant medication.

C. The clinicians often call the managed care company to request fewer sessions.

D. Optimally, the psychotherapist will provide pharmacotherapy without di-
cussing this with the psychopharmacologist.

16.8   Treatment with pharmacotherapy and psychotherapy is a common practice in the
treatment of patients with PDs. Match the *factor* with the best *reason*.

Reason	Factor
A. Medications are generally safer and have more tolerable side effects. Safety is particularly important in a subgroup of PD patients, namely, patients with BPD who have very high suicide rates (Healy 2002).	_____ 1. Managed care plays a significant role.
	_____ 2. Psychopharmacological agents are in more common use today.
B. Companies are often reluctant to approve treatment sessions for patients with PDs who are not receiving pharmacotherapy.	_____ 3. Since the 1990s, there are increased types of psychotherapies for patients with PDs.
C. The nature-nurture dichotomy has been replaced by consideration of the subtle interplay of biological predisposition, resulting in traits that are expressed through behavior that is affected by experiential and environmental factors (Rutter, 2002). Such a theory of interaction between biological and psychological factors and life experience supports a multimodal treatment approach (Paris 1994).	_____ 4. There is a growing appreciation of the role of biological and psychological factors in the etiology of PD symptoms.
D. Treatments such as dialectical behavioral therapy, focused psychotherapy, therapy based on dynamic therapy, interpersonal reconstructive psychotherapy, CBT, and schema-focused CBT.	

The following vignette applies to both questions 16.9 and 16.10:

Mary has been seeing Ms. L, a social worker, for 2 years for trauma she experienced during her military duties and for treatment of BPD. Ms. L sends Mary to see her primary care doctor for medication but does not talk with the doctor ahead of time. When the doctor sees Mary, she believes Mary is getting too dependent on Ms. L. The doctor also surmises that Ms. L is encouraging Mary to leave her current position because of a reenactment of the abuse she felt in the military.

16.9 What might be the best course of action on the part of the primary care doctor?

    A. Request that Mary stop seeing Ms. L.
    B. Request that Mary take an antipsychotic medication.
    C. Call Ms. L, with Mary's permission, and discuss the issues and treatment plan.
    D. Do nothing as Mary's psychotherapy is not a concern for her primary care physician.

16.10 What is a reasonable transference response that Mary might experience upon being referred to the primary care doctor for medication?

    A. Ms. L enjoys caring for Mary.
    B. The psychotherapy with Ms. L is not working.
    C. The primary care doctor is a psychiatrist.
    D. Ms. L is closing her practice.

CHAPTER 17

Boundary Issues

17.1   A 34-year-old woman with dependent personality is being treated in psychodynamic psychotherapy by a male therapist. Which of the following therapist actions is most likely to be a boundary violation?

A. Handing her a tissue when she starts to cry.
B. Answering the patient's question about the therapist's marital status.
C. Setting up a brief phone session between appointments.
D. Asking the patient to bring him coffee when she comes for a session.
E. Sending her a postcard while on a prolonged vacation.

17.2   When a boundary crossing occurs in therapy, it is essential to first do which of the following?

A. Discuss with the patient at the next available occasion.
B. Apologize to the patient at the next session.
C. Only discuss it if the patient brings it up at the next session.
D. Transfer the patient to another therapist.
E. Emphasize to the patient that this is considered a normal part of therapy.

17.3   A male therapist justifies a sexual relationship with a female patient by stating, "It's not my fault—I was seduced." This is not a valid excuse for which of the following reasons?

A. Financial duty.
B. Power asymmetry.
C. Confidentiality.
D. Context dependence.
E. Setting.

17.4   Intrinsic consequences of boundary violations may include which of the following?

A. Ethics complaint to the professional society.
B. Civil lawsuit.
C. Board of registration complaint.
D. Criminal lawsuit.
E. Patient suicide.

17.5 Malpractice insurance will always pay for legal fees involved in which of the following?

A. Any malpractice lawsuit.
B. Any malpractice lawsuit other than for a sexualized boundary violation.
C. Any board of registration complaint other than for a sexualized boundary violation.
D. Ethics complaints.
E. Any board of registration complaint.

17.6 A 39-year-old woman with histrionic personality disorder (PD) tries unsuccessfully to get her therapist to give her a hug. At the end of the session, the therapist walks her to the door and closes it after she leaves. A minute later, the patient starts knocking on the door and loudly calling the therapist's name. An appropriate response might be which of the following?

A. Bringing the patient back into the office and thoroughly discussing her behavior and the reason for acting this way.
B. Telling the patient that if she does not stop this behavior, therapy will need to be terminated.
C. Telling the patient that this behavior is inappropriate and should be discussed at the next session.
D. Bringing the patient back into the office and discussing transfer to another therapist.
E. Calling security to escort the patient out and then calling and referring her to another clinic.

17.7 A female therapist is treating a 29-year-old man with antisocial PD. The most likely indication that the therapist has committed a boundary violation is which of the following?

A. The patient has started calling the therapist by her first name.
B. The therapist has started the patient on an antidepressant.
C. The therapist has volunteered to testify at a parole hearing for the patient.
D. The patient has developed a maternal transference toward the therapist.
E. The patient is demanding to be placed on alprazolam for anxiety.

17.8 Which of the following is defined as the "red flag" that should alert a therapist of an impending boundary violation with a patient who has borderline PD (BPD)?

A. The therapist's realization that an exception to his or her usual practice is about to be made.
B. The patient's sense of entitlement and of being "special."
C. A history of early sexual trauma in the patient.
D. The therapist's recognition of the patient's unconscious manipulation.
E. Recognition of "borderline rage" in a patient.

17.9 Which of the following is the least common cause of boundary transgressions in patients with BPD?

A. The patient's high suicidal risk.
B. Countertransference hostility.
C. The "golden fantasy" entertained by some patients.
D. Countertransference wish to rescue the patient.
E. The patient's excessive familiarity and pseudo-closeness with treaters.

17.10 During which of the following times in therapy are boundary issues more likely to emerge in embryonic form?

A. When the patient and therapist first enter the room and the patient sits down.
B. When medication management is discussed.
C. At the beginning of therapy.
D. When the therapy has ended and the patient is moving toward the door.
E. In the middle of the therapy session.

17.11 If the therapist believes that a boundary crossing may have occurred, what are the next immediate steps?

A. Maintain professional behavior, document, and discharge the patient.
B. Maintain professional behavior, document, and consult with a lawyer.
C. Discuss with the patient, maintain professional behavior, and document.
D. Apologize to the patient, transfer the patient, and document.
E. Discuss with the patient, transfer the patient, and maintain professional behavior.

CHAPTER 18

Assessing and Managing Suicide Risk

18.1 In the "acute-on-chronic" risk model for suicidality in personality disorders (PDs), which of the following is considered an acute risk?

A. Childhood sexual abuse.
B. Poor employment history.
C. Multiple prior treaters.
D. Discharge from the hospital.
E. Low socioeconomic status.

18.2 In DSM-5, the diagnostic criteria of recurrent suicidal or self-injurious behaviors are included in which of the following diagnoses?

A. Paranoid PD.
B. All PDs.
C. Antisocial PD.
D. Borderline PD (BPD).
E. Narcissistic PD.

18.3 What is the estimated lifetime risk of completed suicide for patients with BPD?

A. Substantially less than the other Cluster B PDs.
B. Higher among patients receiving regular outpatient treatment.
C. Between 3% and 10%, depending on the study.
D. About equal to the rate of attempted suicide in BPD.
E. Consistently an 8% rate in all studies.

18.4 Research on suicidality in patients with BPD has indicated the possibility of two patient groups with distinct patterns over time: a group with repeated high-lethality attempts and a group with repeated low-lethality attempts. The group with repeated low-lethality attempts is notable for which of the following?

A. Older age.
B. More psychiatric hospitalizations.

C. Comorbid histrionic or narcissistic PDs.

D. Poor baseline psychosocial functioning.

E. Recruitment for studies from inpatient populations.

18.5   Which of the following is the best description of the stress-diathesis causal model of suicidal behavior?

A. A model suggesting an underlying neurobiologic vulnerability to suicidal behavior in times of stress.

B. Another way to assess and communicate risk of suicide in clinical situations in the acute-on-chronic model.

C. A theory specifically discounting a patient's core personality traits.

D. A model for suicidal behavior developed exclusively for patients with PDs.

E. A model for suicide to be assessed only in retrospective studies.

18.6   Crisis management and safety planning for patients with BPD would likely include which of the following?

A. The intervention developed by Stanley and Brown (2012) to facilitate hospitalization of at-risk patients.

B. Use of a variety of interventions with psychotropic medications except for antipsychotics.

C. Avoidance of involvement with family members as part of crisis intervention.

D. Neuroimaging studies.

E. Patient and clinician's collaborative assessment of suicide risk over time.

18.7   Which of the following best describes the changes over time for patients with BPD?

A. Patients with BPD are not likely to show remission of symptoms of the disorder over time.

B. Patients with BPD are likely to show remission of diagnostic criteria for the disorder over time.

C. Patients with BPD will likely have an increased rate of suicide attempts over time.

D. Patients with BPD are more likely to have increasingly impaired social functioning and improved vocational functioning over time.

E. Patients with a history of childhood sexual abuse and BPD will have fewer suicide attempts over time.

18.8   Health care providers treating suicidal patients with PDs are likely to experience which of the following?

A. Understandable pessimism given data that evidence-based therapies available are not effective in preventing suicidal behavior.

B. Reassurance given the low prevalence of suicidal behavior and death by suicide.

C. Increased concern in cases of recurrent serious suicide attempts.

D. More concern about the risk of suicide for patients with Cluster A or Cluster C disorders than for patients with Cluster B disorder.

E. Optimism when treating patients with antisocial PD given the low rates of suicide in this population.

18.9 What are the findings of studies defining the structural, metabolic, and functional biology of brain circuits mediating personality traits in subjects at high risk for suicidal behavior?

A. Hippocampal volume gain in structural magnetic resonance imaging (MRI) studies of patients with BPD.

B. Increased gray matter concentrations of attempters compared with non-attempters in insular cortex.

C. Improved executive cognitive functioning in borderline subjects under stress leading to suicidal behavior.

D. Excessive cortical inhibition in functional MRI (fMRI) studies of subjects with BPD.

E. Hyperarousal of the amygdala and other limbic structures in fMRI studies of subjects with BPD.

18.10 Which statistic accurately reflects the prevalence and rates of morbidity and mortality associated with PD diagnoses?

A. The prevalence of PDs from the National Comorbidity Survey Replication of approximately 9% of the general population.

B. An estimation that 5% of psychiatric inpatients meet criteria for BPD.

C. An estimation that 20% of psychiatric outpatients meet criteria for BPD.

D. The estimated lifetime rate of attempted suicide of 25% in patients with BPD.

E. Approximately 36% of men and 33% of women in one psychological autopsy study of completed suicide meeting criteria for at least one PD.

C H A P T E R   1 9

Substance Use Disorders

19.1 What is the estimated prevalence of alcohol use disorders in patients with DSM-IV personality disorders (PDs)?

A. 10%.
B. 20%.
C. 30%.
D. 40%.
E. 50%.

19.2 What is the estimated prevalence of drug use disorders in patients with DSM-IV PDs?

A. 10%.
B. 20%.
C. 30%.
D. 40%.
E. 50%.

19.3 Which of the following PDs is classified as an "externalizing disorder"?

A. Avoidant.
B. Schizotypal.
C. Antisocial.
D. Schizoid.
E. Paranoid.

19.4 On what should the treatment focus during the initial phase of psychotherapy with a patient with a dual diagnosis of PD and substance use disorder?

A. Confronting and challenging maladaptive traits.
B. Cognitive-affective processes.
C. Transference/countertransference.
D. Establishment and maintenance of abstinence.
E. Interpersonal relationships.

19.5   Which of the following types of treatment is most useful in patients with dual diagnosis of substance use disorder and PD?

   A. Dialectical behavioral therapy.
   B. Cognitive-behavioral therapy.
   C. Psychodynamic psychotherapy.
   D. Motivational interviewing.
   E. Supportive psychotherapy plus Alcoholics Anonymous.

19.6   Which of the following pharmacotherapies is generally contraindicated in patients with comorbid PDs and substance abuse disorders?

   A. Neuroleptics.
   B. Benzodiazepines.
   C. Selective serotonin reuptake inhibitors (SSRIs).
   D. Lithium.
   E. Buspirone.

19.7   The causal pathway explaining the high comorbidity between substance use disorders and PDs, which suggests that PDs *contribute* to the development of substance use, is known as which of the following?

   A. The behavioral disinhibition pathway.
   B. The stress reduction pathway.
   C. The reward sensitivity pathway.
   D. The primary PD model.
   E. The common factor model.

19.8   Which of the following PDs when comorbid with a substance use disorder predicts the best outcome with a modified version of DBT, known as DBT-S?

   A. Borderline.
   B. Antisocial.
   C. Obsessive-compulsive.
   D. Narcissistic.
   E. Schizotypal.

19.9   Which of the following best describes the difference between DSM-IV and DSM-5 when describing substance abuse versus dependence?

   A. In DSM-IV, substance abuse and substance dependence are a single disorder.
   B. In DSM-5, substance abuse and substance dependence are a single disorder.
   C. In DSM-IV, the presence of tolerance and withdrawal are not criteria that differentiate substance dependence from substance abuse.
   D. In DSM-5, the presence of tolerance and withdrawal are criteria that did not differentiate substance dependence from substance abuse.
   E. There are no differences in the DSM-IV and DSM-5 criteria for substance abuse and substance dependence.

19.10 Which of the following PDs is *not* more prevalent among patients with substance use disorders?

    A. Borderline.
    B. Antisocial.
    C. Obsessive-compulsive.
    D. Narcissistic.
    E. Schizotypal.

CHAPTER 20

Antisocial Personality Disorder and Other Antisocial Behavior

20.1 What do epidemiologic studies reveal about women with antisocial personality disorder (ASPD)?

A. Those who have children have fewer children than do non-antisocial women.
B. They engage in more sexual misbehavior than do their male counterparts.
C. They are as likely as boys to have engaged in fighting, use of weapons, cruelty to animals, or setting fires.
D. Women and men have an equal prevalence of ASPD.
E. They marry at an older age than do their non-antisocial peers.

20.2 What are common attributes of people with ASPD?

A. They generally show remorse after involvement in negative activity.
B. They fail to learn from the negative results of their behavior.
C. They show typical empathy for those negatively affected by their behavior.
D. They often manifest micropsychotic episodes.
E. Their symptomatology rarely presents before age 18 years.

20.3 What does epidemiologic evidence reveal about children with conduct disorder?

A. The prevalence of conduct disorder is evenly distributed between boys and girls.
B. An estimated 50% of girls eventually develop ASPD.
C. An estimated 75% of boys eventually develop ASPD.
D. By age 11 years, 80% of future cases have had a first symptom.
E. The disorder affects approximately 45% of children in the general population.

20.4 What differences between men and women did the National Epidemiologic Survey on Alcohol and Related Conditions (NESARC) study of antisocial personality symptoms show?

A. Men were more likely than women to be deceitful.
B. Men were more likely than women to be impulsive and fail to plan ahead.
C. Men were more likely than women to consistently be irresponsible.
D. Men were more likely than women to lack remorse for their harmful actions.
E. Men were more likely than women to be reckless.

20.5 Which mainstay pharmacologic treatment appears to be the most effective and well supported in the literature when treating ASPD?

A. Risperidone 0.5–2 mg qd.
B. Naltrexone 50 mg qd.
C. Lamotrigine 100–200 mg qd.
D. Clonazepam 0.5–1.5 mg bid.
E. Treatment, if offered, is targeted to any associated mood-substance-related issues.

20.6 Which of the following correctly describes ASPD?

A. Misbehaviors seen in ASPD tend to improve with age.
B. Married individuals with ASPD are more symptomatic than those that are unmarried.
C. ASPD has not been linked to an increased risk for mood disorder.
D. ASPD is not associated with an increased risk of substance abuse.
E. As the etiology of ASPD is biochemical, family factors play little role in the development of ASPD.

20.7 Which of the following is thought to be a risk factor for the development of ASPD?

A. Low rates (2%–4%) of electroencephalographic abnormalities.
B. Possessing a high-activity variant of the MAOA gene.
C. Having antisocial siblings.
D. As children, being cared for by multiple caretakers.
E. An increased volume of prefrontal gray matter.

20.8 What abnormal pathophysiology is associated with ASPD?

A. Low cortisol levels.
B. High testosterone levels.
C. An elevated startle response.
D. Smaller ventricles on neuroimaging.
E. A low resting pulse rate and low skin conductance.

20.9   Which of the following should be included in the differential diagnosis of ASPD?

A. BPD.
B. Obsessive-compulsive disorder.
C. Generalized anxiety disorder.
D. Pervasive developmental disorder.
E. Complicated grief.

20.10 Which of the following is difficult to distinguish from conduct disorder in the evaluation of a child?

A. Oppositional defiant disorder.
B. Posttraumatic stress disorder.
C. Normal development.
D. Adjustment disorder with mixed emotional features.
E. Separation anxiety disorder.

20.11 What is the most well studied and effective mode of psychotherapy in ASPD?

A. Psychoanalysis.
B. Group therapy.
C. Interpersonal therapy.
D. Applied behavioral analysis.
E. There are insufficient data to assess the value of psychotherapy in persons with ASPD.

CHAPTER 21

Personality Disorders in the Medical Setting

21.1 Which of the following is particularly indicative of personality dysfunction in a medical outpatient?

A. A patient who is experienced as "difficult."
B. Disruptive behaviors that have persisted over many years.
C. Unacceptable behavior by a patient recently given a distressing diagnosis.
D. Clinic staff liking the patient very much.
E. A patient who carefully researches the medical diagnosis.

21.2 Research on patients with borderline PD (BPD) in the medical setting indicates that which of the following are common behaviors?

A. Seductive approaches to the clinic staff.
B. Life-threatening remarks to the clinic staff.
C. Unusual openness and willingness to talk with the clinic staff.
D. Yelling and screaming at the clinic staff.
E. Frequent compliments about the clinic to family.

21.3 Which PD is most closely correlated with intentional sabotage of medical care?

A. Paranoid PD.
B. Dependent PD.
C. Avoidant PD.
D. BPD.
E. Schizotypal PD.

21.4 An obstetrical colleague stops you in the hallway to ask about a patient she recently admitted for a nonhealing wound following an emergency caesarean section several weeks ago. She asks, "Could she be intentionally trying to not let the wound heal?" The patient uses only acetaminophen for pain but is demanding that the nursing staff get her special foods. What is the most likely PD diagnosis for this patient?

A. Antisocial.
B. Paranoid.
C. Narcissistic.
D. Borderline.
E. Dependent.

21.5 In what situation would the "Headlines Test" be useful for a primary care physician taking care of a patient?

A. When referring the patient for a psychiatric consultation.
B. When confronting the patient about provocative dress.
C. When telling the patient to stop offering free tickets to the clinic staff.
D. When using the state's online program to check if the patient is obtaining controlled substances from several different physicians.
E. When accepting the patient's invitation to see the Kentucky Derby in the family's private box.

21.6 Which of the following statements correctly describes the relationship between chronic pain and PDs?

A. Younger patients with BPD are more likely to report chronic pain than older patients with BPD.
B. Patients with BPD rarely report chronic pain syndromes.
C. Medical disability is considerably higher in chronic pain patients with BPD compared with those without PD.
D. Medical disability is considerably lower in chronic pain patients with BPD compared with those without PD.
E. Medical disability is no different in chronic pain patients with BPD compared with those without PD.

21.7 What is the goal for the psychiatric consultant for a patient with a PD who is disruptive and uncooperative during an acute medical admission?

A. Engage the patient in psychotherapy to treat the PD.
B. Focus on the unit staff having problematic interactions with the patient to elucidate what is realistically problematic about his or her behavior.
C. Avoid the use of psychotropic medication at all costs.
D. Stabilize the patient in order to complete the medical evaluation and necessary treatment.
E. Take as long as it is necessary to assess the situation and arrive at a plan.

21.8 Which of the following personal physician characteristics may cause unintentional problems in treating patients with PDs in the longitudinal patient-care situation?

A. A physician who is psychosocially minded.
B. Personal physician characteristics have no impact on the relationship with patients who have PDs.

C. A physician who has a clear concept of his or her personal responsibility in the clinical outcome.

D. A physician who shows no response to a patient's intense emotions and passively withdraws from the patient.

E. A physician who feels comfortable with what is and what is not appropriate patient behavior.

21.9 What is the role of the clinician's experience in medicine in dealing effectively with patients who have PDs?

A. Early-career physicians deal more effectively with these patients than do experienced physicians.

B. The idealization of the practice of medicine common early in a physician's career aids in effective management of patients with PDs.

C. The clinical impasses that occur with these patients do not bother early-career physicians.

D. More experienced physicians are less susceptible to unrealistic expectations of themselves and are better able to handle the difficulties involved in treating patients with PDs.

E. Experience does not influence how physicians handle the difficulties involved in treating patients with PDs.

21.10 An internal medicine colleague asks to talk to you about a patient she has followed for 5 years. She recognized at the beginning of treatment that her patient had BPD from the patient's history of chaotic relationships, cutting behaviors, substance abuse, and impulsivity; however, she felt she could manage the patient because her medical condition was one in which the physician was an expert. She has seen the patient biweekly, usually for short visits. Over the past 6 months, she has seen the patient weekly for 30- to 60-minute visits, during which they discuss the patient's relationships. She feels she approaches the patient calmly, even when the patient is unreasonable and monitors for when the patient is seeking extra analgesics or discusses pursuing therapies that might be harmful medically. When the patient has been disruptive in the clinic, the physician has worked with her and the staff to resolve the issues, even though the staff has wanted the patient to be discharged from the clinic. During the 5 years of treatment, the patient complained about the internist's vacations, but last month while the internist was away, the patient cut herself and required stitches to repair the wound. In reviewing the case, what is the mistake that the internist is making in the management of this patient?

A. Attempting to do psychotherapy with the patient.

B. Not discharging the patient from the clinic.

C. Discussing the patient's seeking potentially harmful medical treatments.

D. Involving multiple physicians in the patient's care.

E. Seeing the patient biweekly for many years.

CHAPTER 22

Personality Disorders in the Military Operational Environment

22.1 Which of the following statements about military service is true?

    A. Military leaders are not required to attempt to correct deficiencies and rehabilitate behavior that is detrimental to occupational and social functioning within the military.

    B. Establishment of a diagnosis of a personality disorder (PD) after enlistment is viewed as a condition that did not exist prior to enlistment.

    C. Behavioral health care is not available to military personnel with PDs.

    D. The military does not allow for relatively expeditious administrative separation of service members with PDs.

    E. Stressors in military life may precipitate episodes of decompensation in service members with PDs.

22.2 Which of the following statements concerning medical and psychological screening for enlistment to military service is true?

    A. The U.S. military conducts formal, comprehensive psychiatric and psychological screening tests on all persons entering active military service.

    B. PD diagnoses documented prior to entry into the military serve as bars to enlistment.

    C. Specialized military occupations (e.g., Special Forces) are prohibited from using formal psychological screening for enlistment and selection.

    D. Complete psychological/psychiatric histories are always obtained during the enlistment process.

    E. Prevalence rates for military personnel with PDs are well established and can be used to guide enlistment.

22.3 Which of the following is NOT a standard pathway to mental health care for active duty service members with personality disorders?

A. Service members may obtain a primary care referral to see a mental health specialist.
B. Service members with PDs may self-refer for behavioral health care.
C. Commanders or supervisors may encourage service members to seek mental health treatment.
D. Peers may refer or accompany fellow service members to behavioral health care.
E. All service members receive behavioral health care as a standard component of their medical care.

22.4 Systematic health surveillance studies conducted by the Mental Health Advisory Team (MHAT) during combat operations in Iraq and Afghanistan demonstrated a significant increase in the prevalence of which of the following diagnoses during and after deployment when compared with garrison or predeployment rates?

A. Major depression, substance use disorders, and posttraumatic stress disorder (PTSD).
B. PTSD, substance use disorders, and psychotic disorders.
C. PDs, PTSD, and substance use disorders.
D. Major depression, substance use disorders, and psychotic disorders.
E. Substance use disorders, PDs, and major depression.

22.5 Systematic examination of military health care utilization revealed that incidence rates of which diagnoses remained generally stable or declined between the years 2000 and 2011?

A. Substance use disorders and adjustment disorders.
B. Psychotic disorders and PDs.
C. Adjustment disorders and PTSD.
D. PDs and anxiety disorders.
E. Major depression and adjustment disorders.

22.6 Conditions that render a service member *unsuitable* for military service differ from conditions that render a service member *unfit* for military service in which of the following ways?

A. The terms *unsuitable* and *unfit* are interchangeable designations that do not affect benefits after separation from the military.
B. Determining a service member *unsuitable* for military service allows for medical retirement with benefits.
C. Determining a service member *unfit* for military service may result in administrative separation without benefits.
D. Conditions that can render a service member *unsuitable* for military service include PDs, enuresis, motion sickness, and sleepwalking.
E. Conditions that can render a service member *unfit* for military service include PDs, enuresis, motion sickness, and sleepwalking.

22.7 Who makes the final disposition about a service member's administrative separation from service?

A. A military psychiatrist.
B. A military court-martial.
C. The service member's commander.
D. A Medical Evaluation Board.
E. The service member.

22.8 Recommendations from the Army Task Force on Behavioral Health led to which changes in disability evaluations in military service members in 2011?

A. They allowed disability evaluations to consider behavioral changes that might stem from PDs or adjustment disorders to be eligible solely for administrative separation instead of medical disability compensation.
B. They allowed disability evaluations to consider behavioral changes that may stem from trauma and combat to be eligible solely for administrative separation instead of medical disability compensation.
C. They designated specific guidelines about the conducting of psychological evaluations.
D. They discontinued all administrative separations for behavioral changes in active duty members.
E. They allowed disability evaluations to consider behavioral changes that might stem from PDs and adjustment disorders to be considered in a light that would be most beneficial to the service member in terms of potential disability compensation instead of administrative separation.

22.9 Which of the following diagnostic categories has sufficient overlap of symptoms with PD symptoms, potentially leading to the misdiagnosis and administrative separation of military service members?

A. Traumatic brain injury.
B. Schizophrenia.
C. Sleep-wake cycle disorders.
D. Bereavement.
E. Major depression.

CHAPTER 23

Translational Research in Borderline Personality Disorder

23.1 Which of the following phenotypes of borderline personality disorder (BPD) described by Gunderson and colleagues is its most distinctive and pathogenic component?

A. Antisocial traits.
B. Self-loathing.
C. Interpersonal hypersensitivity.
D. Rejection projection.
E. Provider idealization.

23.2 Research studies have demonstrated that unresolved attachment in BPD has a positive relation to activation in which of the following areas of the brain in response to adult attachment projective images?

A. Amygdala and hippocampus.
B. Visual cortex.
C. Auditory cortex.
D. Frontal lobe.
E. Occipital lobe.

23.3 *Cognitive empathy*, the capacity to take the perspective of another person, and *affective empathy*, the ability to label one's own emotion in the context of emotionally charged situations, have been studied using various research methodologies. In comparison with healthy subjects, cognitive and affective empathy are found at what level in patients with BPD?

A. Cognitive empathy is consistently lower.
B. Affective empathy is consistently lower.
C. Both types of empathy are lower.
D. Both types of empathy are higher.
E. Both types of empathy are the same.

23.4   What is the phenomenon called when a person with BPD is affected by his or her own emotions that are triggered through the emotions of others?

A. Emotional triggering.
B. Emotional contagion.
C. Projective identification.
D. Regressive identity.
E. Reaction formation.

23.5   Which of the following hormones plays a critical role in intimate relationships as well as most meaningful interpersonal relationships?

A. Thyroxine.
B. Estrogen.
C. Testosterone.
D. Oxytocin.
E. Epinephrine.

23.6   Which of the following hormones or neurotransmitters has been found in reduced concentrations in blood samples from women with BPD?

A. Progesterone.
B. Estrogen.
C. Oxytocin.
D. Norepinephrine.
E. Epinephrine.

23.7   Patients with BPD often invoke which of the following type of actions in order to achieve quick release from aversive inner tension?

A. Yelling.
B. Sobbing.
C. Lying.
D. Crying.
E. Cutting.

23.8   In addition to achieving quick release from inner tension, patients with BPD also utilize NSSI to help them accomplish which of the following?

A. Express anxiety and despair.
B. Punish their family and others.
C. Avoid feeling physical pain.
D. Terminate symptoms of dissociation.
E. Act on suicidal feelings.

23.9 Reduction in pain sensitivity in individuals with BPD is an alteration of which pain-processing aspect?

A. Subjective.
B. Affective.
C. Sensory.
D. Spatial.
E. Temporal.

23.10 Patients with dissociative identity disorder demonstrate which of the following neurobiological characteristics?

A. Increased P300 amplitudes.
B. Normal cortical excitability.
C. Normal magnetoencephalography-measured brain waves.
D. Increased pain sensitivity.
E. Reduced volumes of hippocampus and amygdala.

CHAPTER 24

An Alternative Model for Personality Disorders

DSM-5 Section III and Beyond

24.1   Which of the following is the most reasonable critique of the approach taken by DSM-III and DSM-IV to the diagnosis of personality disorders (PDs)?

A. The disorders have too little overlap, not allowing for multiple diagnoses.
B. The criteria allow for the possibility for a wide variety of presentations of the same disorder.
C. The thresholds between normal and pathological were arbitrary.
D. The diagnoses are so rigid as to not allow for symptomatic changes over time.
E. The diagnoses are overinclusive, leaving little room for unique pathological presentations.

24.2   Which of the following explanations is suggested by this observation? The DSM-IV diagnosis of PD not otherwise specified (PDNOS) in DSM-IV-TR is the most commonly diagnosed PD.

A. The diagnoses inadequately cover the possible range of personality pathology.
B. The diagnoses as written are not reliable.
C. The diagnoses are too confusing for most clinicians to use.
D. The diagnoses lack empirical research supporting their validity.
E. PDs cannot be diagnosed using a categorical approach.

24.3   Which of the following best characterizes the DSM-5 "alternative" attempt in Section III, "Emerging Measures and Models" (American Psychiatric Association 2013), to incorporate both dimensional and categorical elements in the PD diagnoses?

A. Hybrid.
B. Polythetic.
C. Monothetic.
D. Categorical.
E. Dimensional.

24.4 In the DSM-5 alternative model for PDs, there are new general criteria for the disorders and pathological personality traits and specific criteria for each individual diagnosis. Which of the following are patients required to demonstrate?

A. Criteria for one of 10 possible PDs.
B. Impairment in personality functioning.
C. Evidence for childhood precursors of their disorder.
D. Comorbidity with an Axis I disorder.
E. Such primitive defenses as splitting or projective identification.

24.5 DSM-IV-TR general criteria for PDs described an enduring pattern of inner experience and behavior that is potentially manifest by affectivity, interpersonal functioning, impulse control, and/or which of the following?

A. Cognition.
B. Pathological personality traits.
C. Disturbances in identity.
D. Difficulties with self-direction.
E. Lack of capacity for intimacy.

24.6 Which of the following has been found to distinguish avoidant PD from social phobia?

A. More problems with self-esteem.
B. Persistent difficulties in social situations.
C. Inability to perform certain tasks (i.e., eating) in public venues.
D. Lack of response to behavioral interventions.
E. Greater likelihood of assigning negative attributes and emotions to others.

24.7 The DSM-5 Section III model for personality traits was derived from which of the following models of personality?

A. Eysenck's three-factor model.
B. Costa and Widiger's five-factor model.
C. Zukerman and Kulman's alternative five model.
D. Hippocrates's four temperaments.
E. Myers Briggs Type Indicator.

24.8 The DSM-5 Section III model describes higher-order trait domains and facets for each domain. The two higher-order trait domains most relevant to antisocial PD are Disinhibition and which of the following domains?

A. Negative affectivity.
B. Detachment.
C. Antagonism.
D. Psychoticism.
E. Neuroticism.

24.9 The DSM-5 Section III model description for borderline personality disorder (BPD) and antisocial PD overlap for which of the following trait facets?

A. Hostility.
B. Manipulativeness.
C. Deceitfulness.
D. Callousness.
E. Grandiosity.

24.10 A person who is high in neuroticism is likely to be described in which of the following ways?

A. Anxious.
B. Oriented toward others.
C. Introverted.
D. Eschewing novelty.
E. Disorderly.

24.11 Which of the following summarizes one of the strongest arguments for using dimensional rather than categorical approaches when diagnosing PDs?

A. Categorical approaches are neither practical nor user friendly.
B. Diagnostic schemes using categorical approaches have an inherent theoretical bias.
C. Differences between normal and pathological personality are ones of degree, not kind.
D. Categorical approaches do not allow for polythetic approaches.
E. There is little interrater reliability with categorical diagnoses.

24.12 Which of the following PDs has the most extensive empirical evidence for validity and clinical utility?

A. Paranoid PD.
B. Schizoid PD.
C. BPD.
D. Histrionic PD.
E. PDNOS.

24.13 Which of the following PDs has the fewest empirical studies supporting their validity?

A. Antisocial PD.
B. Paranoid PD.
C. BPD.
D. Schizotypal PD.
E. Depressive PD.

24.14 Which of the following is most typical of polythetic approaches to diagnoses?

   A. Considers all members of the diagnostic group identical on all characteristics.
   B. Includes broad sets of criteria that are neither necessary nor sufficient.
   C. Makes a clear distinction between normal and pathological.
   D. Considers symptoms on a continuum between normal and pathological.
   E. Incorporates both categorical and dimensional approaches.

24.15 The DSM-5 Section III criteria differ from those of the DSM-IV in that antisocial PD can be diagnosed in the absence of which of the following?

   A. A pervasive pattern of disregard for the rights of others.
   B. A history of childhood conduct disorder.
   C. Violation of the rights of others.
   D. Age of at least 18 years.
   E. Lack of remorse or indifference to hurting others.

24.16 In the DSM-5 Section III, diagnosis of personality disorder–trait specified (PD-TS) differs from PDNOS in that it requires which of the following?

   A. The individual must meet the general criteria for a PD.
   B. The individual cannot meet the criteria for any specific PD.
   C. The individual's symptoms are consistent with a specific pattern of symptoms not included among the accepted PDs.
   D. The specific maladaptive traits should be listed as part of the diagnosis.
   E. The individual meets criteria for more than one PD.

24.17 Schizotypal PD differs from the other DSM-5 Section III disorders in that it includes dysfunction in which of the following domains?

   A. Negative Affectivity.
   B. Detachment.
   C. Antagonism.
   D. Disinhibition versus compulsivity.
   E. Psychoticism.

Part II

Answer Guide

CHAPTER 1

Personality Disorders: Recent History and New Directions

1.1 In the Collaborative Longitudinal Personality Disorders Study (CLPS), what percentage of patients meeting criteria for borderline personality disorder (BPD) at intake showed remission at 10-year follow-up?

A. 15%.
B. 35%.
C. 50%.
D. 65%.
E. 85%.

The correct response is option E: 85%.

Although one of the generic defining features of personality disorders (PDs) is their enduring nature, personality pathology is often activated or intensified by circumstance, such as loss of a job or the end of a meaningful relationship. In the CLPS, stability of DSM-IV–defined PD diagnoses reflected sustained pathology at or above the diagnostic threshold, but substantial percentages of patients showed fluctuation over time, sometimes being above and sometimes below the diagnostic threshold. In the CLPS, which used a stringent definition of remission (the presence of no more than two criteria for at least 1 year), 85% of patients with DSM-IV–defined BPD at intake showed remission at the 10-year follow-up point. **(pp. 7–8)**

1.2 The second edition of the DSM aimed to introduce what major diagnostic concept to the way that PDs were conceptualized and described?

A. Diagnoses aimed to capture constellations of personality that were observable, measurable, enduring, and consistent over time.
B. Diagnoses made based on degree of social and occupational dysfunction.

81

C. Diagnoses reflected evolving and controversial psychoanalytic theories of the time.
D. Diagnoses focused on etiology and pathogenesis of symptoms.
E. Diagnoses clarified degree to which symptoms caused emotional suffering.

The correct response is option A: Diagnoses aimed to capture constellations of personality that were observable, measurable, enduring, and consistent over time.

The first edition of the DSM represented a largely psychoanalytically oriented system of terminology for classifying mental illness precipitated by stress (Barton 1987). The primary stimulus leading to the development of a new, second edition of the DSM was the publication of the eighth edition of the International Classification of Diseases (World Health Organization 1967) and the wish of the American Psychiatric Association (APA) to reconcile its diagnostic terminology with this international system. In the DSM revision process, an effort was made to move away from theory-derived diagnoses and to attempt to reach consensus on the main constellations of personality that were observable, measurable, enduring, and consistent over time. **(pp. 2–4)**

1.3   In DSM-III, what characteristic difference was thought to exist between Axis I and Axis II disorders, which allowed for the separation of the PDs from many other psychiatric illnesses?

A. Axis II disorders were thought to be less severe than Axis I disorders.
B. Axis II disorders were thought to be less genetically determined than Axis I disorders.
C. Axis II disorders were composed of persistent conditions versus the episodic disorders of Axis I.
D. Axis II disorders were derived from psychoanalytic theory, whereas Axis I disorders were empirically based.
E. Axis II disorders were thought to respond to therapy, whereas Axis I disorders were thought to respond to medications.

The correct response is option C: Axis II disorders were composed of persistent conditions versus the episodic disorders of Axis I.

DSM-III defined PDs (and all other disorders) by explicit diagnostic criteria and introduced a multiaxial evaluation system. Disorders classified on Axis I included those generally seen as episodic "symptom disorders" characterized by exacerbations and remissions, such as psychoses, mood disorders, and anxiety disorders. Axis II was established to include the PDs as well as specific developmental disorders; both groups were seen as composed of early-onset, persistent conditions. The decision to place the PDs on Axis II led to greater recognition of the PDs and stimulated extensive research and progress in our understanding of these conditions. In general, DSM III shifted PD diagnosis and understanding away from being psychoanalytically based and toward empirical, symptom-driven assessments. There was no true differentiation between severity of Axis I and Axis II diagnoses, nor was treatment specifically differentiated between medication and therapy, in large part because medication management at the time was far less sophisticated than its current state. **(p. 4)**

1.4　In the transition from DSM-II to DSM-III, schizoid PD was subcategorized into which three PDs?

A. Schizoid, schizotypal, passive-aggressive.
B. Schizoid, schizotypal, avoidant.
C. Schizotypal, borderline, avoidant.
D. Schizotypal, borderline, narcissistic.
E. Schizoid, narcissistic, passive-aggressive.

The correct response is option B: Schizoid, schizotypal, avoidant.

Schizoid PD was felt to be too broad a category in DSM-II, and it was crafted into three PDs in DSM-III: schizoid PD, reflecting "loners" who are uninterested in close personal relationships; schizotypal PD, understood to be on the schizophrenia spectrum of disorders and characterized by eccentric beliefs and nontraditional behavior; and avoidant PD, typified by self-imposed interpersonal isolation driven by self-consciousness and anxiety. BPD and narcissistic PD were both added to the DSM-III. Passive-aggressive PD, as defined by DSM-III and DSM-III-R, was thought to be too unidimensional and generic; it was tentatively retitled "negativistic PD," and the criteria were revised. **(pp. 4–5)**

1.5　In the first edition of DSM, what clinical picture did "personality pattern disturbances" describe?

A. Innate, genetically based features of personality that are present from birth.
B. Conditions that in the absence of stress were not particularly pervasive and disabling.
C. Entrenched conditions likely to be recalcitrant to change.
D. Social deviance behaviors such as sexual deviations, addictions, and antisocial reaction.
E. Episodic personality changes due to mood and psychotic episodes.

The correct response is option C: Entrenched conditions likely to be recalcitrant to change.

In the first edition of the DSM, PDs were generally viewed as deficit conditions, reflecting partial developmental arrests or distortions in development secondary to inadequate or pathological early caretaking (option A). The PDs were grouped primarily into "personality pattern," "personality trait," and "sociopathic personality." Personality pattern disturbances were viewed as the most entrenched conditions, likely to be recalcitrant to change even with treatment; these conditions included inadequate personality, schizoid personality, cyclothymic personality, and paranoid personality. Personality trait disturbances were thought to be less pervasive and disabling, so that in the absence of stress these patients could function relatively well (option B). The category of sociopathic personality disturbances reflected what were generally seen as types of social deviance; it included antisocial reaction, dyssocial reaction, sexual deviation, and addiction (option D). In general, personality pattern was thought to be persistent throughout life not episodic in nature (option E). **(pp. 3–4)**

1.6   In DSM-III, the work of multiple scholars of personality and emotional disturbances significantly influenced and shaped the emergence of what two PD descriptions?

A. Borderline and narcissistic.
B. Borderline and histrionic.
C. Narcissistic and schizotypal.
D. Histrionic and antisocial.
E. Schizotypal and antisocial.

The correct response is option A: Borderline and narcissistic.

Two new PD diagnoses were added in DSM-III: BPD and narcissistic PD. In contrast to initial notions that patients called "borderline" were on the border between the psychoses and the neuroses, the criteria defining BPD in DSM-III emphasized emotional dysregulation, unstable interpersonal relationships, and loss of impulse control more than persistent cognitive distortions and marginal reality testing, which were more characteristic of schizotypal PD. Among many scholars whose work greatly influenced and shaped the conceptualization of borderline pathology introduced in DSM-III were Kernberg (1975) and Gunderson (1984). Although others had described concepts of narcissism, the essence of the current views of narcissistic PD emerged from the work of Millon (1969), Kohut (1971), and Kernberg (1975). **(p. 5)**

1.7   Substantiated, evidence-based treatment guidelines exist for which of the following PDs?

A. Histrionic PD.
B. Paranoid PD.
C. Schizoid PD.
D. Antisocial PD.
E. BPD.

The correct response is option E: BPD.

Although personality pathology has been well known for centuries, it is often thought to reflect weakness of character or willfully offensive behavior, produced by faulty upbringing rather than to be a type of "legitimate" psychopathology. In spite of these common attitudes, clinicians have long recognized that patients with personality problems experience significant emotional distress, often accompanied by disabling levels of impairment in social or occupational functioning. General clinical wisdom has guided treatment recommendations for these patients, at least those who seek treatment, plus evidence-based treatment guidelines have been developed for patients with BPD. Patients with paranoid, schizoid, or antisocial patterns of thinking and behaving often do not seek treatment (options B, C, D). There are currently no evidenced-based treatment guidelines for histrionic personality disorder (option A), although these patients may seek out and benefit from multiple treatments. **(p. 2)**

1.8   Reflecting the ongoing debate regarding how to conceptualize, understand, and thus adequately treat PDs, Section III of DSM-5 establishes a hybrid of what two models of diagnoses and classification?

A. Psychological and biological.
B. Cognitive and behavioral.
C. Dimensional and categorical.
D. State and trait.
E. Interpersonal and intrapersonal.

The correct response is option C: Dimensional and categorical.

One prominent controversy of the DSM is whether a dimensional approach or a categorical one is preferred to classify the PDs. In the early 2000s, the APA convened, in collaboration with the National Institute of Mental Health, a series of research conferences to develop an agenda for DSM-5. Shortly thereafter, the APA established a Work Group on Personality and Personality Disorders for DSM-5. It was challenging for the work group to reach a consensus in support of a single dimensional model for the PDs to be used in clinical practice. In the end, a hybrid dimensional and categorical model was proposed, and this model was approved by the APA as an alternative model and placed in Section III of DSM-5. The alternative model includes six specific PDs, plus a seventh diagnosis of *personality disorder—trait specified* that allows description of individual trait profiles of patients with PDs who do not have any of the six specified disorders. In addition, the alternative model involves assignment of level of impairment in functioning, an important additional element of dimensionality when making PD diagnoses. **(p. 7)**

1.9   The organization of PDs into clusters, odd or eccentric; dramatic, emotional, or erratic; and anxious or fearful, reflects what type of diagnostic classification?

A. Etiological.
B. Dimensional.
C. Categorical.
D. Hierarchical.
E. Ontogenetic.

The correct response is option B: Dimensional.

The DSM system is referred to as categorical and is contrasted to any number of systems referred to as dimensional. However, elements of dimensionality already exist in the traditional DSM categorical system, represented by the organization of PDs into Cluster A (odd or eccentric), Cluster B (dramatic, emotional, or erratic), and Cluster C (anxious or fearful). In addition, a patient can just meet the threshold for a PD or can have all of the criteria, presumably a more extreme version of the disorder. **(p. 6)**

References

Barton WE: The History and Influence of the American Psychiatric Association. Washington, DC, American Psychiatric Press, 1987

Gunderson JG: Borderline Personality Disorder. Washington, DC, American Psychiatric Press, 1984

Kernberg O: Borderline Conditions and Pathological Narcissism. New York, Jason Aronson, 1975

Kohut H: The Analysis of the Self: A Systematic Approach to the Psychoanalytic Treatment of Narcissistic Personality Disorders. New York, International Universities Press, 1971

Millon T: Modern Psychopathology: A Biosocial Approach to Maladaptive Learning and Functioning. Philadelphia, PA, WB Saunders, 1969

World Health Organization: International Classification of Diseases, 8th Revision. Geneva, World Health Organization, 1967

CHAPTER 2

Theories of Personality and Personality Disorders

2.1   Which of the following correctly describes the trait psychological model of personality disorders (PDs)?

A. Trait psychology focuses less than psychodynamic or cognitive-social approaches on personality processes or functions.
B. Trait psychology dichotomizes the pathological and the normal.
C. Trait models define a personality disposition separate from a behavioral tendency.
D. The trait model only incorporates psychodynamic and not biological theory.
E. Trait models of PDs cannot be used to describe clinically derived categories.

The correct response is option A: Trait psychology focuses less than psychodynamic or cognitive-social approaches on personality processes or functions.

The trait psychological model focuses less than psychodynamic or cognitive-social approaches on personality processes or functions and hence has not generated an approach to treatment, although it has generated highly productive empirical research programs. Traits are emotional, cognitive, and behavioral tendencies on which individuals vary (e.g., the tendency to experience negative emotions). Trait theories put the normal and pathological on a spectrum of disorder (option B). An underlying personality disposition is assumed to generate a behavioral tendency (option C). Trait psychological approaches have multiple theoretical underpinnings, including the biological (option D). Lexical analysis of descriptions of personality in *Webster's Unabridged Dictionary* generated the five-factor model (FFM), which is the most prominent contemporary trait theory model. The FFM can be used to translate clinically derived categories into factor language (option E). **(pp. 20–22)**

2.2   What is a key feature of Cloninger's neurobiological model of personality?

A. It divides personality structure into the two domains of temperament and character.
B. It is based on findings from magnetic resonance imaging (MRI) studies.

C. The model does not include a spiritual dimension.

D. The model does not address modes of learning.

E. It defines impulsivity as the major determinant of the presence or absence of PD.

The correct response is option A: It divides personality structure into the two domains of temperament and character.

Cloninger's neurobiological model of personality divides personality structure into two domains: temperament and character. According to Cloninger, these domains are defined by a mode of learning and the underlying neural systems involved in each form of learning (option D). The temperament domain includes four dimensions, each theoretically linked to a particular neurotransmitter system (option B). The character domain includes three dimensions: self-directedness, considered the major determinant of the presence or absence of PD (option E); cooperativeness; and self-transcendence, which includes spirituality, idealism, and enlightenment (option C). **(pp. 22–23)**

2.3   Which idea listed below is a key feature of a psychodynamic point of view of PD?

A. Personality disorders reflect specific pathological symptoms rather than constellations of psychological processes.

B. Personality disorders are the result of the internalization of the attitudes of hostile, abusive, critical, or inconsistent parents and/or significant caretakers.

C. Personality disorders are restricted to a single personality domain.

D. Using the ego psychology model, patients with PDs consistently act in the best interests of others.

E. Patients with PDs can weather momentary failures in the professional arena.

The correct response is option B: Personality disorders are the result of the internalization of the attitudes of hostile, abusive, critical, or inconsistent parents and/or significant caretakers.

Psychoanalytic theorists have turned to the conflict model, ego psychology model, object relations theory, self psychology, and relational theories to help understand patients with PDs. From the ego psychology model comes the insight that people with PDs have various deficits in functioning, such as poor impulse control, difficulty regulating their affects, and deficits in the capacity for self-reflection. These deficits may render them incapable of behaving consistently in their own best interest or taking the interests of others appropriately into account (e.g., lashing out aggressively without forethought, cutting themselves when they become upset) (option D) and reflect processes that are deeply entrenched, which often serve multiple functions and/or have become associated with regulation of affects and are hence resistant to change (option C). Psychoanalytic theorists were the first to generate a concept of PD reflecting the idea that PDs involve character problems not isolated to a specific symptom or set of independent symptoms. From a psychodynamic point of view, they represent constellations of psychological processes, not distinct symptoms that can be understood in isolation (option A). One of the things that distinguishes individuals with PDs from people with healthier character structure is their difficulty weathering momentary failures in the personal or the professional arena (option E). **(pp. 14–16)**

2.4 Which of the following statements is identified as a feature of the framework of Kernberg's psychodynamic theory of personality and PD?

A. Reality testing is not an important concern.
B. Borderline PD (BPD) in the DSM-5 is equivalent to borderline personality organization as described by Kernberg.
C. More severe personality structure is distinguished by more maladaptive modes of regulating emotions through immature, reality-distorting defenses.
D. Personality-disordered patients are able to generate multifaceted representations of themselves and significant others.
E. The conscious self-representations of narcissistic patients are not grandiose, although the ideal representations are grandiose.

The correct response is option C: More severe personality structure is distinguished by more maladaptive modes of regulating emotions through immature, reality-distorting defenses.

In Kernberg's view, people with severe personality pathology are distinguished from people whose personality is organized at a psychotic level by their relatively intact capacity for reality testing (option A). What distinguishes individuals with severe personality pathology from people with healthier character structures includes their maladaptive modes of regulating emotions and their difficulty forming mature, multifaceted representations of themselves and significant others (option D). This level of severe personality disturbance, which Kernberg calls "borderline personality organization" (Kernberg 1996), shares some features with the DSM diagnosis of BPD. However, borderline personality organization is a broader construct, used to describe people who would be appropriately diagnosed with other PDs according to the DSM, including paranoid, schizotypal, antisocial, and narcissistic (option B). According to Kernberg, individuals with narcissistic PD have both conscious grandiose self-representations and conscious ideal representations (option E). **(pp. 15–16)**

2.5 What is a key feature of cognitive-social theories of PDs?

A. They are based on the idea that learned behaviors are generalized.
B. They assume that personality comprises relatively discrete learned processes that are not situation specific.
C. They do not include skills and competencies.
D. They do not take into account the role of environment but rather favor inherent traits and early life experience in the development of PDs.

E. They include the idea that problems in self-regulation are of particular relevance to severe PDs.

The correct response is option E: They include the idea that problems in self-regulation are of particular relevance to severe PDs.

Of particular relevance to severe PDs is self-regulation, which refers to the process of setting goals and subgoals, evaluating one's performance in meeting these goals, and adjusting one's behavior to achieve these goals in the context of ongoing feedback (Bandura 1986; Mischel 1990). From a behaviorist perspective, personality consists of learned behaviors and emotional reactions that tend to be relatively specific (rather than highly generalized) (option A) and tied to particular environmental contingencies (option B). Cognitive-social theories focus on a number of variables presumed to be most important in understanding PDs, including schemas, expectancies, goals, skills and competencies (option C), and self-regulation (Bandura 1986, 1999; Cantor and Kihlstrom 1987; Mischel 1973, 1979; Mischel and Shoda 1995). Although particular theorists have tended to emphasize one or two of these variables in explaining PDs, such as the schemas involved in encoding and processing information about the self and others (Beck et al. 2004) or the deficits in affect regulation seen in patients with BPD (Linehan 1993b), a comprehensive cognitive-social account of PDs would likely address all of them. From a cognitive-social perspective, personality reflects a constant interplay between environmental demands and the way the individual processes information about the self and the world (Bandura 1986) (option D). **(pp. 17–18)**

2.6   Which of the following is a key element in Linehan's concept of BPD?

A. In contrast to psychodynamic theories, it is silent on the importance of the development of a stable sense of self.
B. It downplays the importance of physiological responses to emotional arousal.
C. It defines a major problem in BPD as a difficulty in inhibiting inappropriate behavior related to intense affect.
D. It considers refocusing of attention as a maladaptive defense mechanism.
E. It downplays the importance of developing interpersonal strategies to the setting of personal goals.

The correct response is option C: It defines a major problem in BPD as a difficulty in inhibiting inappropriate behavior related to intense affect.

The key characteristics of emotion dysregulation in Linehan's (1993a) theory of BPD include difficulty 1) inhibiting inappropriate behavior related to intense affect, 2) organizing oneself to meet behavioral goals (option E), 3) regulating physiological arousal associated with intense emotional arousal (option B), and 4) refocusing attention when emotionally stimulated (option D). Deficits in emotion regulation lead to other problems, such as difficulties with interpersonal functioning and the development of a stable sense of self (option A). **(p. 18)**

2.7 Which of the options below correctly describes a feature of Westen's model of domains of personality functioning?

A. It is based on psychoanalytic theory but not on empirical research.
B. It is a trait model.
C. It requires the use of the Shedler-Westen Assessment Procedure (SWAP-200).
D. It uses insights drawn from many psychoanalytic theoretical schools of thought, including those of ego psychology, self psychology, attachment theory, and object relations theory.
E. It only describes disturbed personality styles and dynamics not healthy personality styles.

The correct response is option D: It uses insights drawn from many psychoanalytic theoretical schools of thought, including those of ego psychology, self psychology, attachment theory, and object relations theory.

Westen has described a model of domains of personality functioning that draws substantially on psychoanalytic clinical theory and observation as well as on empirical research in personality, cognitive, developmental, and clinical psychology (option A). The model is less a theory of PDs than an attempt to delineate and systematize the major elements of personality that define a patient's personality, whether or not the patient has a PD. It shares with trait approaches the view that a single model should be able to accommodate relatively healthy as well as relatively disturbed personality styles and dynamics (option E). The model differs from trait approaches in its focus on personality processes and functions (option B). Westen and Shedler (1999) used this model as a rough theoretical guide to ensure comprehensive coverage of personality domains in developing items for the SWAP-200 Q-sort, a personality pathology measurement for use by expert informants, although the model and the measure are not closely linked (option C). **(pp. 28–29)**

2.8 Benjamin's interpersonal theory of personality is called the Structural Analysis of Social Behavior (SASB). Which of the statements below is a correct description of the model?

A. The SASB is a one-dimensional model.
B. It is a circumflex model in which all three surfaces describe interpersonal patterns.
C. It is a model capable of specifying the interpersonal antecedents that elicit a patient's responses.
D. It is a model that aims to specify a single motivation to explain a behavior.
E. It is unrelated to the PD diagnoses as described in the DSM.

The correct response is option C: It is a model capable of specifying the interpersonal antecedents that elicit a patient's responses.

Benjamin's SASB focuses on interpersonal processes in personality and psychopathology and their intrapsychic causes, correlates, and sequelae. It is influenced by Sullivan's (1953) interpersonal theory, object relations approaches, and research. The SASB is a three-dimensional model, with three "surfaces" (option A). The first surface focuses on actions directed at another person. A second surface focuses on the person's response to real or perceived actions by the other. The third focus is on the person's actions toward himself or herself, or what Benjamin calls the "introject" (option B). The SASB offers a translation of each of the DSM-IV PD criteria and disorders into interpersonal terms (option E). The SASB model is able to represent multiple, often conflicting aspects of the way patients with a given disorder behave (or complex, multifaceted aspects of a single interpersonal interaction) simultaneously (option D). **(pp. 27–28)**

2.9   Which statement below correctly describes the utility of behavioral genetic approaches to PDs?

A. They address the lack of consensus among trait psychologists regarding which traits to study by studying the causes of trait covariation.
B. They preferentially study abnormal personality traits found in PDs rather than normal personality traits.
C. They direct twin and adoption studies that demonstrate consistent and precise heritability of PDs.
D. They demonstrate that the heritability of PDs is less than 20%.
E. They show that BPD is primarily biologically determined.

The correct response is option A: They address the lack of consensus among trait psychologists regarding which traits to study by studying the causes of trait covariation.

Compared with research on adaptive personality traits, behavioral genetic studies of PDs are less common (option B). As in all behavioral genetic research, twin and adoption studies provide more definitive data. The results have often showed significant variability (option C), most likely due to the range of samples and the methods used. Although the precise heritability estimate may vary, several PDs have consistently shown heritability figures in the 0.40–0.60 range or above (option D). The majority of studies have examined only a few DSM PDs. These disorders appear to reflect a continuum of heritability, with schizotypal most strongly linked to genetic influences; antisocial linked both to environmental and genetic variables; and borderline showing the smallest estimates of heritability in the majority of studies (option E). **(pp. 24–26)**

2.10   Early maladaptive schemas (EMSs) are an augmentation of cognitive-behavioral personality theory promulgated by Young to address aspects of personality development, which take place at a young age. Which statement about EMS below is correct?

A. It is an extension of Kohut's theories of the grandiose self.
B. Young believes that schema maintenance, schema avoidance, and schema compensation are the three most important cognitive processes involving schemas that define key features of PDs.
C. Young's theories are incompatible with psychodynamic and attachment theories.
D. EMSs equate with automatic thoughts and underlying assumptions.
E. Young has identified 10 EMSs.

The correct response is option B: Young believes that schema maintenance, schema avoidance, and schema compensation are the three most important cognitive processes involving schemas that define key features of PDs.

Building on Beck's cognitive theory (option A), Young has added a fourth level of cognition, EMSs, defined as "broad and pervasive themes regarding oneself and ones relationships with others, developed during childhood and elaborated throughout one's life" (Young and Lindemann 2002, p. 95). More recently, Young and colleagues have incorporated psychodynamic and attachment theories, and some strategies from emotion-focused approaches, resulting in a more integrative conceptualization and treatment of PDs (option C). Young distinguishes these from automatic thoughts and underlying assumptions (option D), noting that early maladaptive schemas are associated with greater levels of affect, are more pervasive, and involve a strong interpersonal aspect. Young and colleagues have identified 18 EMSs, each comprising cognitive, affective, and behavioral components (option E). **(p. 19)**

References

Bandura A: Social Foundations of Thought and Action. Englewood Cliffs, NJ, Prentice-Hall, 1986
Bandura A: Social cognitive theory of personality, in Handbook of Personality: Theory and Research, 2nd Edition. Edited by Pervin L, John O. New York, Guilford, 1999, pp 154–196
Beck A, Freeman A, Davis D: Cognitive Therapy of Personality Disorders, 2nd Edition. New York, Guilford, 2004
Cantor N, Kihlstrom JF: Personality and Social Intelligence. Englewood Cliffs, NJ, Prentice-Hall, 1987
Kernberg O: A psychoanalytic theory of personality disorders, in Major Theories of Personality Disorder. Edited by Clarkin J, Lenzenweger M. New York, Guilford, 1996, pp 106–140
Linehan M: Cognitive-Behavioral Treatment of Borderline Personality Disorder. New York, Guilford, 1993a
Linehan M: Skills-Training Manual for Treatment of Borderline Personality Disorder. New York, Guilford, 1993b
Mischel W: Toward a cognitive social learning reconceptualization of personality. Psychol Rev 39:351–364, 1973 4721473
Mischel W: On the interface of cognition and personality: beyond the person-situation debate. Am Psychol 34:740–754, 1979
Mischel W: Personality dispositions revisited and revised: a view after three decades, in Handbook of Personality: Theory and Research. Edited by Pervin L. New York, Guilford, 1990, pp 111–134

Mischel W, Shoda Y: A cognitive-affective system theory of personality: reconceptualizing situations, dispositions, dynamics, and invariance in personality structure. Psychol Rev 102:246–268, 1995 7740090

Sullivan HS: The Interpersonal Theory of Psychiatry. New York, WW Norton, 1953

Westen D, Shedler J: Revising and assessing Axis II, part 1: developing a clinically and empirically valid assessment method. Am J Psychiatry 156:258–272, 1999 9989563

Young J, Lindemann M: An integrative schema-focused model for personality disorders, in Clinical Advances in Cognitive Psychotherapy: Theory and Application. Edited by Leahy R, Dowd T. New York, Springer, 2002, pp 93–109

CHAPTER 3

Articulating a Core Dimension of Personality Pathology

3.1 The DSM-5 Personality and Personality Disorders Work Group proposed that core impairments found in personality disorders (PDs) should be assessed using a dimensional approach. Which of the following clinicians might have disagreed with using a dimensional approach to assessing psychopathology?

A. Sir Francis Galton.
B. Emil Kraepelin.
C. Otto Kernberg.
D. Jean Piaget.
E. J.C. Prichard.

The correct response is option B: Emil Kraepelin.

Emil Kraepelin delineated classes of disorders such as manic-depression and dementia praecox that were presented as qualitatively different phenomenon, whereas many personality-oriented writers (including Sir Francis Galton, Otto Kernberg, Jean Piaget, and J.C. Prichard) continued to emphasize a more unitary (dimensional) approach that identified critical differences as existing between points along a single continuum. **(p. 41)**

3.2 A number of reliable and valid measures exist for assessing personality functioning and psychopathology. Which of the following measures provides a dimensional assessment of identity, primitive defenses, and reality testing and is based upon a model of personality advanced by Kernberg?

A. General Assessment of Personality Disorder (GAPD).
B. Severity Indices of Personality Problems (SIPP).
C. Social Cognition and Object Relations Scale (SCORS).
D. Structured Interview of Personality Organization (STIPO).
E. Thematic Apperception Test (TAT).

The correct response is option D: Structured Interview of Personality Organization (STIPO).

The STIPO is a semistructured interview based on a model of personality health and disorder advanced by Kernberg (Kernberg 1984; Kernberg and Caligor 2005). Questions were designed to provide a dimensional assessment of identity, primitive defenses, and reality testing, which help clinicians determine the level of disorder in personality functioning. The GAPD, SIPP, and SCORS were all designed to assess dimensions of self and interpersonal functioning but were not based upon Kernberg's model of personality organization. The TAT is a projective psychological test. **(pp. 43–44)**

3.3   In the literature review conducted by Bender et al. (2011), which of the following rubrics captured components most central to effective personality functioning?

A. Identity, self-direction, empathy, intimacy.
B. Reality testing, defensive structure, object representations, self representations.
C. Cognition, libido, affective lability, impulse control.
D. Obsessionality, hysteria, masochism, narcissism.
E. Mood, anxiety, psychosis, substance use.

The correct response is option A: Identity, self-direction, empathy, intimacy.

Bender et al. (2011) found that the components most central to effective personality functioning fall under the rubrics of identity, self-direction, empathy, and intimacy, with reliability estimates for measures of these constructs typically exceeding 0.75. Reality testing, defensive structure, and self/other object representations are components that determine level of personality functioning (option B) as described by Kernberg. Obsessionality, hysteria, masochism, and narcissism are character styles or traits (option D). Mood, anxiety, psychosis, and substance use are general categories of psychiatric disorders found in DSM-5 (option E). Cognition, libido, affect lability, and impulse control are a random assortment of terms (option C). **(p. 44)**

3.4   Mary meets seven of nine criteria for borderline PD (BPD), whereas Andrea meets five of nine criteria for BPD. Which of the following is likely to be a true statement about each person?

A. Andrea is more likely than Mary to meet criteria for additional PDs.
B. Mary is more likely than Andrea to meet criteria for additional PDs.
C. Andrea is more likely than Mary to have a history of childhood trauma.
D. Mary is more likely than Andrea to have a history of childhood trauma.
E. There is not any meaningful difference between Mary and Andrea's likelihood of comorbidity or history of trauma.

The correct response is option B: Mary is more likely than Andrea to meet criteria for additional PDs.

Widiger et al. (1989) found that "prototypical" patients who met all criteria for a PD were more likely than "average" patients (who only met some of the criteria for a PD) to have additional PD diagnoses. **(pp. 44–45)**

3.5 The Level of Personality Functioning Scale (LPFS; American Psychiatric Association, 2013) represents a single-item composite evaluation of impairment in identity, self-direction, empathy, and intimacy. It was designed to serve as a basis for determining global level of impairment in personality functioning in DSM-5. Which of the following is true of the LPFS?

A. It has good sensitivity and good specificity for identifying the presence or absence of DSM-IV PDs.
B. It has good sensitivity but poor specificity for identifying the presence or absence of DSM-IV PDs.
C. It has poor sensitivity but good specificity for identifying the presence or absence of DSM-IV PDs.
D. It has poor sensitivity and poor specificity for identifying the presence or absence of DSM-IV PDs.

The correct response is option A: It has good sensitivity and good specificity for identifying the presence or absence of DSM-IV PDs.

The LPFS has solid sensitivity (0.846) and specificity (0.727) for identifying the presence or absence of DSM-IV PDs. **(pp. 47–48)**

3.6 In which of the following areas did specific PD diagnoses prove useful as a supplement to the LPFS rating of personality impairment?

A. Estimated prognosis.
B. Estimating number of medical comorbidities.
C. Optimal level of treatment intensity.
D. Psychosocial functioning.
E. Risk assessment.

The correct response is option E: Risk assessment.

Morey et al. (2013) conducted analyses to compare the incremental validity of the DSM-5 LPFS rating to DSM-IV PD diagnoses with respect to their ability to predict clinical judgments of psychosocial functioning, short-term risk, estimated prognosis, and optimal level of treatment intensity. All predictive validity correlations for both LPFS ratings and DSM-IV diagnoses were statistically significant. However, results indicated that for three of the four validity variables, the single-item DSM-5 LPFS rating yielded adjusted multiple correlations that were larger than those provided when considering all 10 DSM-IV PD diagnoses. In the areas of functioning, prognosis, and treatment intensity needs (options D, A, and C), the DSM-5 LPFS successfully captured an appreciable part of the valid variance contributed by DSM-IV PD diagnoses and significantly incremented that information as well. Only in the area of risk assessment did information about the specific PD diagnoses prove useful as a supplement to the LPFS rating of impairment in personality functioning. Medical comorbidities (option B) were not considered when exploring predictive validity of LPFS ratings and DSM-IV diagnoses. **(pp. 47–48)**

3.7   Morey et al. (2013) demonstrated that clinicians felt the clinical utility of DSM-IV criteria was more useful than the DSM-5 LPFS rating scale for which of the following?

   A. Communicating to the patient.
   B. Communication with other professionals.
   C. Patient description.
   D. Research studies.
   E. Treatment planning.

The correct response is option B: Communication with other professionals.

Clinicians were asked six questions about perceived clinical utility of each set of information provided. Compared with the DSM-5 LPFS rating, DSM-IV was seen as easier to use and more useful for communication with other professionals. However, in every other respect—for treatment planning, patient description, and communicating to the patient (options E, C, and A)—the DSM-5 LPFS had higher mean usefulness ratings than DSM-IV. Thus, clinicians perceive the single-item DSM-5 LPFS rating as being generally more useful in several important ways than the entire set of 79 DSM-IV PD criteria. This is in spite of these clinicians' presumed greater familiarity with DSM-IV over the past 18 years and their lack of experience with the DSM-5 Section III proposal at the time of the study. The DSM-5 LPFS rating was not compared with DSM-IV criteria in terms of utility for research studies. **(p. 48)**

3.8   Reliable and valid clinician-administered measures of personality functioning and psychopathology generally have a significant focus on which of the following?

   A. Affective lability.
   B. IQ scores.
   C. History of traumatic life events.
   D. Representations of self and other.
   E. Reality testing and perceptual disturbances.

The correct response is option D: Representations of self and other.

In the process of attempting to identify core impairments in personality functioning, Bender et al. (2011) reviewed a number of reliable and valid clinician-administered measures for assessing personality functioning and psychopathology and demonstrated that content relevant to representations of self and other permeates such instruments and that these instruments have solid empirical bases and significant clinical utility. **(p. 43)**

References

American Psychiatric Association: Diagnostic and Statistical Manual of Mental Disorders, 5th Edition. Arlington, VA, American Psychiatric Association, 2013

Bender DS, Morey LC, Skodol AE: Toward a model for assessing level of personality functioning in DSM-5, part I: a review of theory and methods. J Pers Assess 93:332–346, 2011 22804672

Kernberg OF: Severe Personality Disorders: Psychotherapeutic Strategies. New Haven, CT, Yale University Press, 1984

Kernberg OF, Caligor E: A psychoanalytic theory of personality disorders, in Major Theories of Personality Disorder. Edited by Clarkin JF, Lenzenweger MF. New York, Guilford, 2005, pp 114–156

Morey LC, Bender DS, Skodol AE: Validating the proposed DSM-5 severity indicator for personality disorder. J Nerv Ment Dis 201:729–735, 2013 23995027

Widiger TA, Morey LC, Freiman KE: DSMIIIR and DSMIV decision rules for the personality disorders. Paper presented at the meeting of the American Psychological Association, New Orleans, LA, August 1989

CHAPTER 4

Development, Attachment, and Childhood Experiences

4.1 Who formulated the basic tenets of the attachment theory?

A. Mary Ainsworth.
B. John Bowlby.
C. Carol George.
D. Anthony Bateman and Peter Fonagy.
E. Jean Piaget.

The correct response is option B: John Bowlby.

Attachment theory (Bowlby 1969) describes how individuals manage their most intimate relationships with their "attachment figures": their parents, children, and romantic partners. Ainsworth (1978) developed "the most influential protocol for observing individual differences in infants' attachment security," the Strange Situation (option A). George (1994) and Hesse (2008) thereafter came up with the Adult Attachment Interview, which is based on reported attachment narratives of the subject's childhood (option C). Bateman and Fonagy (2006) formulated the mentalization-based theory and treatment of BPD (option D). Piaget (1951) developed the concept of egocentrism (option E). Ainsworth, George, Fonagy, and Piaget did not formulate the basic tenets of the attachment theory. **(pp. 55–56, 66, 68)**

4.2 A child is playing in the room and does not react when the mother leaves the room or when a stranger enters. The child continues to play when the mother returns. The description of this "Strange Situation" is most consistent with which of the following attachment pattern in infants?

A. Anxious/resistant.
B. Securely attached.
C. Disoriented/disorganized.
D. Anxious/preoccupied.
E. Avoidant.

The correct response is option E: Avoidant.

An avoidant infant appears less anxious at separation, may not seek contact with the caregiver on his or her return, and may not seem to prefer the caregiver over the stranger. A child with anxious/resistant attachment (option A) shows less interest in exploration and play in the new environment, becomes highly distressed by the separation, and struggles to settle after being reunited with the caregiver. The securely attached infant (option B) curiously investigates his or her surroundings in the primary caregiver's presence, appears anxious in the stranger's presence, is distressed by the caregiver's brief absence, rapidly seeks contact with the caregiver when the caregiver returns, and is easily reassured enough to resume exploration. The disoriented/disorganized infant (option C) will show undirected or bizarre behavior such as freezing, hand clapping, or head banging or may try to escape the situation. Anxious/preoccupied (option D) describes one of the attachment styles in adults based on the Adult Attachment Interview (AAI). **(p. 56)**

4.3   What is the correlation between infant attachment predicted by the Strange Situation procedure and adult attachment classification based on the AAI?

A. 68%–75%.
B. 5%–15%.
C. 100%.
D. 20%–35%.
E. 75%–90%.

The correct response is option A: 68%–75%.

The correlation in attachment classification between infancy and adulthood is 68%–75%. **(p. 57)**

4.4   Childhood trauma is strongly associated with which of the following personality disorder (PD) and adult attachment style pairs?

A. Schizoid PD and incoherent/disorganized.
B. Borderline PD (BPD) and incoherent/disorganized.
C. Dependent PD and anxious/preoccupied.
D. Antisocial PD and avoidant/ dismissing.
E. Histrionic PD and anxious/preoccupied.

The correct response is option B: Borderline PD (BPD) and incoherent/disorganized.

Childhood trauma is strongly correlated with an incoherent/disorganized adult attachment style more than just to the general category of insecurity. BPD is more consistently associated with childhood abuse and neglect than other PD diagnoses. **(p. 58)**

4.5   In addition to oxytocin, which other neurotransmitter has been shown to play a crucial role in attachment behavior?

A. Serotonin.
B. Anandamide.
C. Dopamine.
D. Substance P.
E. Glutamine.

The correct response is option C: Dopamine.

Two major neural systems have been shown to play a critical role in attachment behaviors: the dopaminergic reward-processing system and the oxytocinergic system (Fonagy et al. 2011). Options A, B, D, and E are incorrect because although each one of them is a neurotransmitter, none has been known to have a major direct involvement in attachment behavior. **(pp. 59–60)**

4.6   What is the effect of oxytocin in the insecurely attached patient with BPD?

A. It increases trust and reduces dysphoric response to social stress.
B. It increases trust but increases dysphoric response to social stress.
C. It does not have any effect on trust in individuals with BPD.
D. It decreases trust but reduces dysphoric response to social stress.
E. It decreases trust and increases dysphoric response to social stress.

The correct response is option D: It decreases trust but reduces dysphoric response to social stress.

Oxytocin acts to neutralize negative feelings toward others and to enhance trust. Secure attachment leads to "adaptive hypoactivity" of the hypothalamic-pituitary-adrenal axis, which, in turn, reduces social anxiety. It must be noted that these positive effects of oxytocin are not universal. In the case of insecurely attached patients with BPD, oxytocin *decreases* trust and the likelihood of cooperative responses, but it reduces dysphoric responses to social stress. **(p. 60)**

4.7   Which of the following is not a key determinant in problematic affect regulation and self-control stemming from dysfunctional attachment relationship?

A. A robust mentalizing capacity.
B. Maltreatment.
C. Failure to develop good interpersonal skills.
D. Failure to self-reflect.
E. High levels of parental mentalization about their children.

The correct response is option A: A robust mentalizing capacity.

Problems in affect regulation, attentional control, and self-control stemming from dysfunctional attachment relationships are mediated through a failure to develop a robust mentalizing capacity. Maltreatment disorganizes the attachment system. There is also evidence to suggest that it may disrupt mentalization (option B). Failure to develop good interpersonal skills may stem from failure to develop a solid mentalizing capacity. Mentalization involves both a self-reflective component and an interpersonal component (options C, D). Parental mentalization about their children, i.e., more reflective parenting practices, including the quality of parental control, parental discourse about emotions, the depth of parental discussion involving affect, parental beliefs about parenting, and non-power-assertive disciplinary strategies that focus on mental states, all help to develop a child's robust mentalization capacity and therefore help with affect regulation and self-control (option E). **(pp. 62–63)**

4.8   Mind-related comments by mothers when a child was 6 months predicted what capacity of the child at 45 and 48 months?

A. IQ scores.
B. Vocabulary.
C. Secure attachment.
D. Imaginary play.
E. Mentalizing.

The correct response is option E: Mentalizing.

Meins and colleagues found that mind-related comments by mothers at 6 months predicted attachment security at 12 months (Meins et al. 2001) and mentalizing capacity at 45 and 48 months (Meins et al. 2002). IQ scores and vocabulary were not part of the latter study's outcomes (options A, B). Mind-related comments by mothers when a child was 6 months predicted attachment security at 12 months (Meins et al. 2001) (option C). Although mentalization is involved in imaginary play, this study did not directly examine imaginary play (option D). **(p. 63)**

4.9   What aspect of child development is explained by the theory of pedagogy?

A. School readiness.
B. Attachment.
C. Tantrums.
D. Subjectivity.
E. Pretend play.

The correct response is option D: Subjectivity.

Young children assume that knowledge of subjective states is also common and that there is nothing unique about their own thoughts or feelings. A sense of the uniqueness of their own perspective develops only gradually. The theory of pedagogy does describe the pattern of learning in infants in children, but it does not focus on school readiness (option A). The quality of attachment plays a role in the acquisition of subjectivity, but the theory of pedagogy does not specifically explain attachment (option B). Pedagogy theory can help us understand why toddlers are more prone to tantrums because they expect everyone to know what they are thinking and feeling. However, this theory does not explain tantrums in general (option C). Although pretend play can help facilitate the development of one's subjectivity and understanding that separate minds have differential content, the theory of pedagogy does not explain pretend play (option E). **(pp. 65–66)**

4.10   Which two adult attachment styles are associated with treatment dropout?

A. Secure and avoidant.
B. Secure and preoccupied.
C. Anxious and disorganized.
D. Avoidant and preoccupied.
E. Secure and disorganized.

The correct response is option D: Avoidant and preoccupied.

Avoidant attachment constitutes a risk for dropout because patients are not fully committed, attached, or engaged with the therapist or the treatment. Preoccupied patients are at risk of dropout after perceived abandonments such as emergency cancellations or scheduled vacations. **(p. 71)**

4.11   In a randomized controlled trial of transference-focused psychotherapy (TFP), dialectical behavior therapy (DBT), and supportive therapy, which treatment modality achieved an increased number of patients classified as secure after treatment?

A. Treatment as usual.
B. TFP.
C. DBT.
D. Supportive therapy.
E. Treatment has no effect on attachment.

The correct response is option B: TFP.

TFP achieved an increased number of patients classified as secure after treatment. None of the other study conditions (options A, C, D, E) showed this outcome. Even though DBT is effective for decreasing impulsive self-harm behaviors in patients with BPD, it did not show an increased number of securely attached patients after treatment (Levy et al. 2006). **(p. 72)**

References

Ainsworth MDS, Blehar MC, Waters E, et al: Patterns of Attachment: A Psychological Study of the Strange Situation. Hillsdale, NJ, Erlbaum, 1978

Bateman A, Fonagy P: Mentalization-Based Treatment for Borderline Personality Disorder: A Practical Guide. New York, Oxford University Press, 2006

Bowlby J: Attachment and Loss, Vol 1: Attachment. London, Hogarth Press and Institute of Psycho-Analysis, 1969

Fonagy P, Luyten P, Strathearn L: Borderline personality disorder, mentalization, and the neurobiology of attachment. Infant Ment Health J 32:47–69, 2011

George C, Kaplan J, Main M: The Adult Attachment Interview. Unpublished manuscript, Department of Psychology, University of California at Berkeley, 1994

Hesse E: The Adult Attachment Interview: protocol, method of analysis, and empirical studies, in Handbook of Attachment: Theory, Research and Clinical Applications, 2nd Edition. Edited by Cassidy J, Shaver PR. New York, Guilford, 2008, pp 395–433

Levy KN, Meehan KB, Kelly KM, et al: Change in attachment patterns and reflective function in a randomized control trial of transference-focused psychotherapy for borderline personality disorder. J Consult Clin Psychol 74:1027–1040, 2006 17154733

Meins E, Fernyhough C, Fradley E, et al: Rethinking maternal sensitivity: mothers' comments on infants' mental processes predict security of attachment at 12 months. J Child Psychol Psychiatry 42:637–648, 2001 11464968

Meins E, Fernyhough C, Wainwright R, et al: Maternal mind-mindedness and attachment security as predictors of theory of mind understanding. Child Dev 73:1715–1726, 2002 12487489

Meins E, Fernyhough C, Wainwright R, et al: Pathways to understanding mind: construct validity and predictive validity of maternal mind-mindedness. Child Dev 74:1194–1211, 2003 12938713

Piaget J: The Child's Conception of the World. London, Routledge/Kegan Paul, 1951

CHAPTER 5

Genetics and Neurobiology

5.1   DSM-5 conceptualizes personality disorders (PDs) in terms of which of the following assessment systems?

A. Dimensional approach.
B. Interacting traits approach.
C. Categorical classification.
D. Interpersonal functioning scale.
E. Impairment-based metrics.

The correct response is option C: Categorical classification.

Although DSM-5 recognizes the value of a dimensional approach and this is acknowledged in Section III, "Emerging Measures and Models," of the DSM-5, the primary system of the DSM for diagnosing the PDs, from DSM-III (American Psychiatric Association 1980) through DSM-5 (American Psychiatric Association 2013), is based on categorical classification. Understanding PDs through interacting traits (option B) is a variation on the dimensional approach (option A) with a long tradition in academic psychology but not yet adopted as the primary system of the DSM-5. Interpersonal functioning and impairment metrics (options D, E) are important across the different diagnoses but do not constitute a classification scheme. **(pp. 79–80)**

5.2   Affective instability, a defining trait of borderline PD (BPD), is associated with changes *primarily* in which of the following affects?

A. Anger, jealousy, shame.
B. Anger, euphoria, guilt.
C. Anger, anxiety, depression.
D. Anger, suspicion, distrust.
E. Anger, disappointment, loneliness.

The correct response is option C: Anger, anxiety, depression.

Although options A, B, D, and E capture moods (euphoria, depression), emotions (jealousy, shame, guilt), cognitive states (suspicion, distrust), and mixed emotion-cognitive states (disappointment, loneliness) that may present in abnormal ways in BPD, the primary affects that demonstrate instability of affect are anger, anxiety, and depression (Koenigsberg et al. 2002). **(p. 80)**

5.3 Which of the following is an empirical finding supporting the notion of heightened sensitivity to emotional stimuli in patients with BPD?

A. A bias to preferentially identify faces with negative or hostile emotions.
B. A need for greater visual information than control subjects.
C. Greater capacity for reallocation of attention than control subjects when faced with affective stimuli.
D. Greater capacity for cognitive reappraisal than control subjects when faced with affective stimuli.
E. Greater reliance on habituation to control highly charged stimuli.

The correct response is option A: A bias to preferentially identify faces with negative or hostile emotions.

Patients with BPD are less accurate overall in identifying emotion in others because they most likely have a bias to preferentially identify negative or hostile emotions (Domes et al. 2009). Reallocation of attention, cognitive reappraisal, and reliance on habituation (options C, D, E) are mechanisms used by healthy persons to control emotional intensity. These mechanisms are believed to be impaired in persons with BPD. Patients with BPD require less visual information than healthy control subjects (option B) to correctly identify facial emotions. **(p. 80)**

5.4 In healthy people, certain brain regions have been paired with particular functions and thus have become regions of interest for assessing PD and other psychopathology. Which of the following is an empirically based pairing of regions and their primary functionality?

A. Rostral anterior cingulate cortex (ACC) and cognitive processing.
B. Insula and motor coordination.
C. Fusiform gyrus and facial recognition.
D. Amygdala and decision making.
E. Dorsal ACC and visual processing.

The correct response is option C: Fusiform gyrus and facial recognition.

The fusiform gyrus is a structure specialized for face processing. The rostral ACC has been implicated in emotion processing (option A) and the dorsal ACC in cognitive processing, cognitive modulation of emotion, and integration of emotional information for adaptively planning behavioral responses (option E). The insula plays an important role in the integration of affective, cognitive, and interoceptive (stimuli within the body) aspects of emotion as well as in emotional appraisal and social emotion (option B). The amygdala is a structure particularly relevant to emotion processing (option D). It is engaged during fear processing as well as during the assessment of emotional salience and in processing facial expressions. **(p. 81)**

5.5   Brain volumes of specific regions, as measured by magnetic resonance imaging (MRI), have shown differences between patients with BPD and healthy control subjects. Which of the following is a consistently reported difference between patients with BPD and healthy control subjects?

A. Smaller amygdala volumes in patients with BPD.
B. Decreased cingulate gray matter volumes in patients with BPD.
C. Decreased anterior cingulate gray matter volumes in female patients with BPD.
D. Increased hippocampus volumes in patients with BPD.
E. Decreased ventral cingulate volumes in patients with BPD, independent of comorbid depression.

The correct response is option B: Decreased cingulate gray matter volumes in patients with BPD.

Patients with BPD have decreased cingulate gray matter (Hazlett et al. 2005; Minzenberg et al. 2008) and hippocampal volumes (option D) (Nunes et al. 2009) relative to healthy control subjects, and this finding has been sustained in meta-analysis (Nunes et al. 2009). Amygdala volumes (option A) in patients with BPD have been reported as increased (Minzenberg et al. 2008), the same (New et al. 2007), and decreased (Brambilla et al. 2004; Driessen et al. 2000; Nunes et al. 2009; Schmahl et al. 2003; Tebartz van Elst et al. 2003). Examining gender differences and correlates of the structural anomalies in BPD, Soloff et al. (2008) found decreased gray matter density in patients with BPD compared with healthy control subjects in the ventral cingulate and in a number of temporal lobe regions, including the amygdala, hippocampus, parahippocampal gyrus, and uncus in both genders. Controlling for the current level of depression, all of these differences remained except the ventral cingulate (option E). Only male patients with BPD showed decreased gray matter concentrations in the ACC (option C) (Soloff et al. 2008). **(pp. 81–82)**

5.6   Difficulties with emotion regulation in patients with BPD have long been recognized. Which of the following is an empirically supported functional MRI (fMRI) finding that supports this clinical observation?

A. Compared with healthy control subjects, patients with BPD showed greater activation of dorsal ACC and intraparietal sulcus in response to attempts to downregulate their responses to disturbing pictures.
B. Compared with healthy control subjects, patients with BPD showed less fusiform face region activity when viewing photographs depicting emotional faces.
C. Compared with healthy control subjects, patients with BPD showed rapid behavioral habituation to negative pictures.

D. Compared with healthy control subjects, patients with BPD showed greater activation of the primary visual areas and the superior temporal gyrus when viewing negative versus neutral pictures.
E. Compared with healthy control subjects, patients with BPD showed a decrease in insular and an increase in orbitofrontal cortex (OFC) activity during attempted distancing.

The correct response is option D: Compared with healthy control subjects, patients with BPD showed greater activation of the primary visual areas and the superior temporal gyrus when viewing negative versus neutral pictures.

When viewing negative pictures compared with neutral pictures, patients with BPD showed greater activation of the primary visual areas and the superior temporal gyrus (Koenigsberg et al. 2009b), indicating greater attention to negative affective stimuli. Similarly, increased amygdala and fusiform face region activity has also been identified in subjects with BPD viewing photographs depicting emotion-inducing scenes (option B) (Herpertz et al. 2001; Koenigsberg et al. 2009b). On the other hand, when it came to controlling these responses, patients with BPD were unable to activate appropriate *control* regions (option C). In an fMRI study in which patients with BPD and healthy control subjects were asked to downregulate their emotional reactions to disturbing pictures by distancing, the patients with BPD were not able to activate the dorsal ACC or intraparietal sulcus, regions implicated in emotion regulation and attentional allocation, to the extent that healthy control subjects did (option A) (Koenigsberg et al. 2009a). In addition, the patients with PD did not decrease insula activity and did not increase orbitofrontal activity (option E) as healthy control subjects did (Schulze et al. 2011). Such processes are highly adaptive and form the basis for desensitization-based psychotherapies. Thus patients with BPD do not engage the same brain regions as healthy control subjects do when attempting to downregulate negative affect using cognitive reappraisal, and they do not downregulate amygdala and insula activity as healthy control subjects do. **(pp. 81–82)**

5.7   Which of the following symptom domains is *least* accounted for by genetic factors?

A. Affective instability.
B. Identity problems.
C. Negative relationships.
D. Avoidance.
E. Self-harm.

The correct response is option E: Self-harm.

A heritability study of the four main symptom domains associated with BPD (affective instability, identity problems, negative relationships, and self-harm) showed that a genetic common pathway model that accounted for 51% of the overall variance best explained heritability. For each BPD scale (options A, B, C), except self-harm, around 50% of its variance was explained by the latent unitary BPD factor (Distel et al. 2010). Avoidance is not one of the four main symptom domains in BPD (option D). **(p. 83)**

5.8   Impulsive aggression plays an important role in the clinical presentation of patients with BPD. Which of the following is true regarding the nature and measurement of this aggression?

   A. Self-reported impulsive aggression remains the best way to distinguish BPD from PD.
   B. The Point Subtraction Aggression Paradigm (PSAP) is an effective behavioral measure of impulsive-aggressive tendencies.
   C. Subjects with high impulsive aggression also showed greater OFC activity during a provocation.
   D. Impulsive aggression is measurable under both provoking and nonprovoking situations.
   E. Impulsive aggression is mostly confined to BPD, being a rare manifestation of another PD.

   The correct response is option B: The Point Subtraction Aggression Paradigm (PSAP) is an effective behavioral measure of impulsive-aggressive tendencies.

   Self-report measures do not distinguish between patients with BPD and patients with other PDs (option A). The PSAP is an effective behavioral measure of the tendency for impulsive aggression that creates a laboratory simulation of frustration and provokes "aggressive" responses; it has been shown to separate healthy control subjects from persons with PD diagnoses. Aggressive responding on the PSAP correlated with symptoms of reactive aggression, and individuals with a high degree of aggression showed impaired recruitment of control mechanisms of the OFC during aggression provocation (option C) (New et al. 2009). Impulsive aggression is present across PDs and only measurable under "provoked" conditions (options D, E). **(pp. 83–84)**

5.9   Impulsive aggression in BPD has been shown to have neurobiological correlates. Which of the following is a neurobiological correlate of impulsive aggression in BPD?

   A. Increased metabolism from serotonergic stimulation with D,L-fenfluramine.
   B. Increased synthesis of serotonin under normal resting conditions.
   C. Adult-onset lesions of the OFC.
   D. Disruption of coupling of the OFC and the amygdala.
   E. Increased brain metabolism in OFC and anterior cingulate gyrus (ACG) in response to meta-chlorophenylpiperazine (mCPP) administration.

   The correct response is option D: Disruption of coupling of the OFC and the amygdala.

Disruption of amygdala-OFC coupling has been shown in patients with BPD with impulsive aggression (New et al. 2007), which is presumed to block the top-down control (OFC) of an intense amygdala (bottom-up) response to a perceived danger signal. A number of studies have demonstrated decreased metabolic activity in OFC and ACG in response to serotonergic challenge in impulsive aggressive patients with BPD compared with healthy control subjects. One study demonstrated that healthy control subjects showed increased metabolism in ACG and OFC following serotonergic stimulation, whereas patients with BPD showed decreased metabolism in these areas (option A) (Soloff et al. 2000). There is no evidence that the synthesis of serotonin under normal resting conditions is lower in BPD (option B). Other work showed reduced metabolic responses after mCPP administration in medial OFC and ACG in impulsive aggressive patients compared with control subjects (option E) (New and Hazlett 2002). Childhood lesions of the OFC (option C) can lead to aggressive behavior in adulthood (Raine and Lencz 2000). **(pp. 84–86)**

5.10 The trust game is a laboratory simulation game that measures "players'" capacity for interpersonal trust. Choose the most accurate statement about the findings on patients with BPD versus healthy control subjects using this laboratory task.

   A. Consistent with rapid overvaluation of others, patients with BPD self-reported greater trust in game partners.
   B. When playing the trustee role, patients with BPD induced distrust in healthy control game partners.
   C. Consistent with interpersonal sensitivity, the anterior insula of patients with BPD demonstrated greater responsivity (than healthy control subjects) to the amount of trust shown toward them.
   D. Patients with BPD tended to underestimate the potential of being taken advantage of in the game.
   E. Despite interpersonal difficulties, the patients with BPD did not become hypervigilant to being taken advantage of in the game.

The correct response is option B: When playing the trustee role, patients with BPD induced distrust in healthy control game partners.

Trust may be studied in the laboratory by means of a multiround economic exchange game, the trust game, in which one participant (the investor) chooses how much money to invest with a trustee. The money is tripled, and the trustee then chooses how much of the current amount to return to the investor. The investor shows trust by the amount he or she invests, and the trustee either reciprocates the trust with generous sharing of profits or maximizes personal short-term gain by keeping most of the profit. The cycle repeats over multiple rounds, allowing for appropriate reciprocal responses. When patients with BPD played this game in the role of trustee interacting with healthy volunteer investors, trust rapidly broke down, as demonstrated by a reduction in the amount invested with a trustee with BPD versus a healthy volunteer trustee (option D) from early to late rounds in the game (King-Casas et al. 2008). Trustees with BPD also self-reported lower levels of trust in the investor than did healthy trustees (option A). The fMRI data reveal that during the time period in each round when healthy trustees learned how much was invested with them, the anterior insula activated in inverse proportion to the amount invested, signaling a perceived feeling of unfairness or violation of social norm. In contrast, trustees with BPD showed a flat insula response (option C), suggesting an anomalous neural response to interpersonal norm violation. Lacking such a natural neural mechanism to monitor interpersonal unfairness, the patient with BPD may resort to a defensive stance, becoming hypervigilant to being taken advantage of (option E). Thus the trust game captures aspects of interpersonal difficulties that patients with BPD demonstrate clinically. (pp. 86–89)

5.11   Which of the following therapies is least likely to treat successfully the interpersonal hypersensitivity associated with patients with BPD?

A. Mentalization-based therapy.
B. Facial emotion-recognition training.
C. Social norm violation awareness training.
D. Desensitization to perceived rejection.
E. Motivational interviewing.

The correct response is option E: Motivational interviewing.

There is evidence of a multifaceted breakdown in social processes in patients with BPD, which could contribute to interpersonal hypersensitivity. Each of the therapies suggested, except motivational interviewing (which has other uses), could possibly address a very specific social process deficit. A better understanding of the social processing disturbances could help shape these treatment strategies to improve the quality of the relationships in the lives of patients with BPD. (pp. 86–89)

5.12   Pain perception in patients with BPD has long been recognized to be anomalous and to be related to self-injurious behaviors. Choose the answer that most correctly pairs an fMRI finding and its clinical correlate.

A. Patients with BPD showed decreased activation of the dorsolateral prefrontal cortex in response to pain and experienced pain as less aversive.
B. Thermal stimuli, acting as an emotional distracter, reduced amygdala response to emotional pictures in patients with BPD but not in healthy control subjects.
C. Patients with BPD showed less signal decrease than healthy control subjects in posterior aspect of the default mode network (DMN) during pain processing, indicating greater self-preoccupation and less aversive experience of the pain.
D. ACC and right amygdala were unchanged in patients with BPD during pain processing, indicating a decreased pain response.
E. Greater connectivity in the DMN system in patients with BPD indicates they overengage emotional regulatory systems.

The correct response is option C: Patients with BPD showed less signal decrease than healthy control subjects in posterior aspect of the default mode network (DMN) during pain processing, indicating greater self-preoccupation and less aversive experience of the pain.

The DMN is a network implicated in internally preoccupied non-task-related processing and in self-referential thinking. Patients with BPD showed less of a signal decrease compared with healthy control subjects in the posterior DMN during pain processing (Kluetsch et al. 2012) (option E). This is consistent with a model in which patients with BPD are more self-preoccupied during the experience of pain, experience pain as less aversive than healthy control subjects do, and do not engage emotion regulatory systems to address the pain to the extent that healthy control subjects do. In addition, when exposed to comparable subjective levels of thermal pain, patients with BPD, relative to healthy control subjects, showed increased activation (option A) of the dorsolateral prefrontal cortex and deactivation of the perigenual ACC and the right amygdala (Schmahl et al. 2006). The ACC is a component of the affective-motivational pain pathway, and the dorsolateral prefrontal cortex has been implicated in pain control. To get at the role of emotional context of pain experience, fMRI images were obtained as subjects were shown emotionally negative pictures in the context of painful or control thermal stimuli. Thermal stimuli, both painful and control, reduced amygdala and insula activity in patients with BPD as well as healthy volunteers (options B, D), suggesting that a nonspecific attentional mechanism decreases limbic activity in response to thermal sensory stimuli (Niedtfeld et al. 2010). **(pp. 89–90)**

5.13   Schizotypal PD (STPD) is characterized by disturbances of many areas including cognition. Choose the statement that most accurately describes the cognitive and associated deficits in STPD.

   A. Cognitive deficits in patients with STPD have similar severity to those found in schizophrenia.
   B. Auditory but not visual memory deficits have been found in patients with STPD.
   C. Smooth pursuit eye movement deficits have been identified in patients with STPD.
   D. Failure of medial frontal pole and anterior frontal pole to compensate for frontal lobe deficits may explain cognitive symptoms in patients with STPD.
   E. P_{50} auditory-evoked potential abnormalities have been shown to differentiate schizophrenia patients from patients with STPD.

The correct response is option C: Smooth pursuit eye movement deficits have been identified in patients with STPD.

A large body of evidence (Siever and Davis 2004) suggests that smooth pursuit eye movements, in particular, are impaired in patients with STPD. The cognitive deficits are less severe in STPD (approximately 1 standard deviation below the mean of healthy control subjects) than in patients with schizophrenia (2 standard deviations below the mean of healthy control subjects) (option A). Moreover, anomalies in P_{50} auditory-evoked potentials have been observed in patients with schizophrenia and STPD (option E) (Siever and Davis 2004). A particular finding of interest in STPD is that frontal lobe–based deficits, specifically those of the dorsolateral prefrontal cortex, may lead to compensatory activity in other frontal regions (option D), such as the medial frontal and anterior frontal pole (Hazlett et al. 2012). Finally, both auditory and visual memory deficits have been found in patients with STPD (option B). **(p. 92)**

5.14   Symptoms profiles in patients with STPD are correlated with neurobiological findings. Choose the correct statement regarding the association of neurobiological findings and symptoms profiles in patients with STPD.

    A. Negative and positive symptoms of STPD are both associated with increased dopamine activity and reversed with dopamine antagonists.

    B. Patients with STPD are better buffered than patients with schizophrenia in regard to subcortical dopamine release provoked by [^{123}I]iodobenzamide (IBZM).

    C. Positron emission tomography (PET) studies indicate a decrease in D_1 receptor availability in STPD, suggesting a mechanism for amphetamine administration in improving the associated cognitive deficits.

    D. D_1 antagonists may enhance cognition in patients with STPD by lowering the excess dopamine activity in the frontal lobes.

    E. The fact that neuroleptics have failed to have an effect on psychotic-like symptoms of STPD has been explained by the negative effects that blocking dopamine activity in these patients may have.

The correct response is option B: Patients with STPD are better buffered than patients with schizophrenia in regard to subcortical dopamine release provoked by [^{123}I]iodobenzamide (IBZM).

Patients with STPD show increased release of dopamine in striatal structures, as indexed by amphetamine-induced displacement of IBZM binding (Abi-Dargham et al. 2004). Evidence suggests that there is a bivariate relationship of dopamine with psychotic-like and deficit-like symptoms, such that increased dopamine activity is related to greater psychotic-like activity, whereas decreased dopaminergic activity is associated with increased deficit-like symptoms (option A) (Roussos and Siever 2012). In studies of dopamine release utilizing IBZM, however, people with STPD do not show the increased release associated with actively psychotic schizophrenia patients (Abi-Dargham et al. 2004). Thus to the extent that patients with STPD are better buffered with respect to subcortical dopaminergic activity, they may be protected against the severe psychosis of schizophrenia. A PET study with the D_1 receptor radioligand [^{11}C]NNC 112 suggested that poorer working memory performance was associated with greater frontal cortical D_1 receptor availability, specifically in patients with STPD (option C) but not in healthy control subjects (Abi-Dargham et al. 2002). According to this hypothesis, people with STPD might respond to D_1 agonists with improvement in working memory owing to their intrinsically low dopaminergic activity in their prefrontal cortex (option D). Moreover, several studies have shown that the symptoms of STPD do respond to neuroleptic medication (option E) (Ripoll et al. 2011). **(pp. 93–94)**

5.15 Social function is impaired in patients with STPD. Choose the correct statement regarding social deficits in patients with STPD.

A. Social anxiety is not qualitatively distinct from the social anxiety in other PDs.
B. Smooth pursuit eye movement deficits correlate with social difficulties in healthy control subjects.
C. Facial emotion-cognition failed to correlate with social anxiety in healthy control subjects.
D. The social anxiety of a patient with STPD will attenuate as he or she becomes familiar with particular individuals or social situations.
E. Patients with STPD report concerns that they will be rejected as the driving cognition behind their anxiety.

The correct response is option B: Smooth pursuit eye movement deficits correlate with social difficulties in healthy control subjects.

In a study of healthy control subjects, those selected by virtue of their impaired smooth pursuit eye movement tended to have fewer friends, had more trouble or discomfort in dating, and were uncomfortable socially. These characteristics were more clearly associated with inaccuracy of the smooth pursuit system than the psychotic-like symptoms of STPD (Siever and Davis 2004). Thus impaired cortical information processing can impede the development of accurate, empathic representations of others and can interfere with the interpretation of interpersonal cues. Although anxiety occurring in social contexts is common in other PDs (e.g., avoidant), there are important qualitative distinctions from what occurs in patients with STPD (option A). For example, social anxiety in STPD tends not to attenuate with familiarity with other persons or with greater experience within a particular social context (option D). In other patients with PDs with social anxiety but not in patients with STPD, there are more specific and characteristic feared interpersonal situations or associated maladaptive beliefs (option E). A recent study, however, demonstrated a correlation between impaired facial affect recognition and schizotypal spectrum social anxiety in healthy individuals (option C) assessed with the Schizotypal Personality Questionnaire (Abbott and Green 2013). **(pp. 95–96)**

5.16 Antisocial PD (ASPD) and psychopathy have long been recognized as different but overlapping concepts. Choose the correct statement regarding differences between these conditions.

A. Psychopaths show greater difficulty identifying fear in facial emotion tasks than patients with ASPD.

B. On an emotional version of a go/no-go task, patients with psychopathy showed blunted processing of negative emotional words, whereas patients with ASPD showed appropriate processing of negative emotional words regardless of inhibitory control demands.

C. Both patients with psychopathy and patients with ASPD demonstrate aggression of the instrumental (strategic) type.

D. Executive functioning, which is responsible for behavioral control in healthy control subjects, is significantly impaired in patients with ASPD and even more so in patients with psychopathy.

E. Patients with ASPD and patients with psychopathy have similar findings on frontal imaging studies.

The correct response is option B: On an emotional version of a go/no-go task, patients with psychopathy showed blunted processing of negative emotional words, whereas patients with ASPD showed appropriate processing of negative emotional words regardless of inhibitory control demands.

Event-related brain potentials were studied during a go/no-go task in offenders with psychopathy, offenders with ASPD, and a control group of offenders. In the control group, inhibitory control demands modulated frontal P3 amplitude to negative emotional words, indicating appropriate prioritization of inhibition over emotional processing. In contrast, the psychopathic group showed blunted processing of negative emotional words regardless of inhibitory control demands (Verona et al. 2012). A meta-anaylsis showed substantial deficits in fear recognition in subjects with ASPD, and this was consistent regardless of the absence or presence of psychopathy (option A) (Marsh and Blair 2008). Individuals with ASPD engage in aggressive behavior that is more retaliatory/impulsive (i.e., road rage) rather than instrumental (option C). Impulsive aggression reflects a lack of impulse control (Dolan and Park 2002), whereas individuals with psychopathy often engage in strategic instrumental violence. Although the data strongly support a disruption of amygdala and prefrontal cortex functioning—specifically, in the OFC, ACG, and dorsolateral prefrontal cortex—in individuals with psychopathic traits and/or antisocial behavior, the data for ASPD itself (option E) are less conclusive (Nordstrom et al. 2011; Yang et al. 2009). A large meta-analysis of 39 studies found that although *antisocial behaviors* and *psychopathic features* were associated with executive dysfunction, executive function deficits among subjects with ASPD were statistically significant but of such a minor degree as to be clinically imperceptible (option D), and others could find no differences in executive function between ASPD and healthy or psychiatric control subjects (Morgan and Lilienfeld 2000). **(pp. 96–98)** Antisocial Personality Disorder

References

Abbott GR, Green MJ: Facial affect recognition and schizotypal personality characteristics. Early Interv Psychiatry 7:58–63, 2013 22369486

Abi-Dargham A, Mawlawi O, Lombardo I, et al: Prefrontal dopamine D1 receptors and working memory in schizophrenia. J Neurosci 22:3708–3719, 2002 11978847

Abi-Dargham A, Kegeles LS, Zea-Ponce Y, et al: Striatal amphetamine-induced dopamine release in patients with schizotypal personality disorder studied with single photon emission computed tomography and [123I]iodobenzamide. Biol Psychiatry 55:1001–1006, 2004 15121484

American Psychiatric Association: Diagnostic and Statistical Manual of Mental Disorders, 3rd Edition. Washington, DC, American Psychiatric Association, 1980

American Psychiatric Association: Diagnostic and Statistical Manual of Mental Disorders, 5th Edition. Arlington, VA, American Psychiatric Association, 2013

Brambilla P, Soloff PH, Sala M, et al: Anatomical MRI study of borderline personality disorder patients. Psychiatry Res 131:125–133, 2004 15313519

Distel MA, Willemsen G, Ligthart L, et al: Genetic covariance structure of the four main features of borderline personality disorder. J Pers Disord 24:427–444, 2010 20695804

Dolan M, Park I: The neuropsychology of antisocial personality disorder. Psychol Med 32:417–427, 2002 11989987

Domes G, Schulze L, Herpertz S: Emotion recognition in borderline personality disorder—a review of the literature. J Pers Disord 23:6–19, 2009 19267658

Driessen M, Herrmann J, Stahl K, et al: Magnetic resonance imaging volumes of the hippocampus and the amygdala in women with borderline personality disorder and early traumatization. Arch Gen Psychiatry 57:1115–1122, 2000 11115325

Hazlett EA, New AS, Newmark R, et al: Reduced anterior and posterior cingulate gray matter in borderline personality disorder. Biol Psychiatry 58:614–623, 2005 15993861

Hazlett EA, Goldstein KE, Kolaitis JC: A review of structural MRI and diffusion tensor imaging in schizotypal personality disorder. Curr Psychiatry Rep 14:70–78, 2012 22006127

Herpertz SC, Dietrich TM, Wenning B, et al: Evidence of abnormal amygdala functioning in borderline personality disorder: a functional MRI study. Biol Psychiatry 50:292–298, 2001 11522264

King-Casas B, Sharp C, Lomax-Bream L, et al: The rupture and repair of cooperation in borderline personality disorder. Science 321:806–810, 2008 18687957

Kluetsch RC, Schmahl C, Niedtfeld I, et al: Alterations in default mode network connectivity during pain processing in borderline personality disorder. Arch Gen Psychiatry 69:993–1002, 2012 22637967

Koenigsberg HW, Harvey PD, Mitropoulou V, et al: Characterizing affective instability in borderline personality disorder. Am J Psychiatry 159:784–788, 2002 11986132

Koenigsberg HW, Fan J, Ochsner KN, et al: Neural correlates of the use of psychological distancing to regulate responses to negative social cues: a study of patients with borderline personality disorder. Biol Psychiatry 66:854–863, 2009a 19651401

Koenigsberg HW, Siever LJ, Lee H, et al: Neural correlates of emotion processing in borderline personality disorder. Psychiatry Res Neuroimaging 172:192–199, 2009b 19394205

Marsh AA, Blair RJ: Deficits in facial affect recognition among antisocial populations: a meta-analysis. Neurosci Biobehav Rev 32:454–465, 2008 17915324

Minzenberg MJ, Fan J, New AS, et al: Frontolimbic structural changes in borderline personality disorder. J Psychiatr Res 42:727–733, 2008 17825840

Morgan AB, Lilienfeld SO: A meta-analytic review of the relation between antisocial behavior and neuropsychological measures of executive function. Clin Psychol Rev 20:113–136, 2000 10660831

New AS, Hazlett EA: Blunted prefrontal cortical 18fluorodeoxyglucose positron emission tomography response to meta-chlorophenylpiperazine in impulsive aggression. Arch Gen Psychiatry 59:621–629, 2002 12090815

New AS, Hazlett EA, Buchsbaum MS, et al: Amygdala-prefrontal disconnection in borderline personality disorder. Neuropsychopharmacology 32:1629–1640, 2007 17203018

New AS, Hazlett EA, Newmark RE, et al: Laboratory induced aggression: a positron emission tomography study of aggressive individuals with borderline personality disorder. Biol Psychiatry 66:1107–1114, 2009 19748078

Niedtfeld I, Schulze L, Kirsch P, et al: Affect regulation and pain in borderline personality disorder: a possible link to the understanding of self-injury. Biol Psychiatry 68:383–391, 2010 20537612

Nordstrom BR, Gao Y, Glenn AL, et al: Neurocriminology, in Advances in Genetics. Edited by Huber R, Bannasch DL, Brennan P. New York, Academic Press, 2011, pp 255–283

Nunes PM, Wenzel A, Borges KT, et al: Volumes of the hippocampus and amygdala in patients with borderline personality disorder: a meta-analysis. J Pers Disord 23:333–345, 2009 19663654

Raine A, Lencz T: Reduced prefrontal gray matter volume and reduced autonomic activity in antisocial personality disorder. Arch Gen Psychiatry 57:119–127, 2000 10665614

Ripoll LH, Triebwasser J, Siever LJ: Evidence-based pharmacotherapy for personality disorders. Int J Neuropsychopharmacol 14:1257–1288, 2011 21320390

Roussos P, Siever LJ: Neurobiological contributions, in Oxford Handbook of Personality Disorders. Edited by Widiger T. New York, Oxford University Press, 2012, pp 299–324

Schmahl CG, Vermetten E, Elzinga BM, et al: Magnetic resonance imaging of hippocampal and amygdala volume in women with childhood abuse and borderline personality disorder. Psychiatry Res 122:193–198, 2003 12694893

Schmahl C, Bohus M, Esposito F, et al: Neural correlates of antinociception in borderline personality disorder. Arch Gen Psychiatry 63:659–667, 2006 16754839

Schulze L, Domes G, Kruger A, et al: Neuronal correlates of cognitive reappraisal in borderline patients with affective instability. Biol Psychiatry 69:564–573, 2011 21195392

Siever LJ, Davis KL: The pathophysiology of schizophrenia disorders: perspectives from the spectrum. Am J Psychiatry 161:398–413, 2004 14992962

Soloff PH, Meltzer CC, Greer PJ, et al: A fenfluramine-activated FDG-PET study of borderline personality disorder. Biol Psychiatry 47:540–547, 2000 10715360

Soloff PH, Nutche J, Goradia D, et al: Structural brain abnormalities in borderline personality disorder: a voxel-based morphometry study. Psychiatry Res 164:223–236, 2008 19019636

Tebartz van Elst L, Hesslinger B, Thiel T, et al: Frontolimbic brain abnormalities in patients with borderline personality disorder: a volumetric magnetic resonance imaging study. Biol Psychiatry 54:163–171, 2003 12873806

Verona E, Sprague J, Sadeh N: Inhibitory control and negative emotional processing in psychopathy and antisocial personality disorder. J Abnorm Psychol 121:498–510, 2012 22288907

Yang Y, Raine A, Narr KL, et al: Localization of deformations within the amygdala in individuals with psychopathy. Arch Gen Psychiatry 66:986–994, 2009 19736355

CHAPTER 6

Prevalence, Sociodemographics, and Functional Impairment

6.1   In the general population, what is the approximate prevalence for any personality disorder (PD)?

A. <1%.
B. Between 1% and 2%.
C. Between 3% and 5%.
D. Between 10% and 15%.
E. Between 20% and 25%.

The correct response is option D: Between 10% and 15%.

The prevalence rate for any PD is very similar across studies, with the majority of studies finding a prevalence of between 10% and 15% in the general population. On average, the prevalence rates of specific PDs are around 1.5%. Cluster C PDs are most prevalent with a rate around 7.0%, whereas the prevalence rates for Cluster A and Cluster B are approximately 3.5%. **(p. 112)**

6.2   Which PD occurs most frequently in the general population?

A. Antisocial PD.
B. Borderline PD (BPD).
C. Dependent PD.
D. Narcissistic PD.
E. Obsessive-compulsive PD.

The correct response is option E: Obsessive-compulsive PD.

With a rate of around 2.5%, avoidant and obsessive-compulsive PDs are the most frequent PDs affecting the general population. Although there are variations in the prevalence rates found by studies, the rank order or the relative frequency of occurrence in the general population is relatively consistent. BPD (option B) and antisocial PD (option A) come next and affect approximately 1.5% of the population each. Dependent PD (option C) affects approximately 1% of the population, and many studies find <1% prevalence rates for narcissistic PD (option D). **(p. 112)**

6.3   How do point prevalence rates of PDs change over a lifetime?

A. Rates increase as the population ages.
B. Rates decrease as the population ages.
C. Rates are mostly constant as the population ages.
D. Rates vary unpredictably as the population ages.
E. Rates increase until age 50 and then decrease.

The correct response is option C: Rates are mostly constant as the population ages.

The study by Johnson et al. (2008) of adolescents followed from age 14 years to 32 years found that the mean point prevalence of PDs over four observation points—14, 16, 22, and 33 years—was 13.4%. The cumulative prevalence over the four time points was 28.2%. Given the empirical research that shows that many treated individuals are free of their PDs after a relatively short time (Grilo et al. 2004; Shea et al. 2002; Skodol et al. 2005; Zanarini et al. 2006), it is implied that new cases have to debut in the population to replace those that disappear, even if some reappear (Durbin and Klein 2006; Ferro et al. 1998; Zanarini et al. 2006). **(pp. 113–114)**

6.4   Which PD is much more prevalent in the clinical population than in the general population?

A. BPD.
B. Obsessive-compulsive PD.
C. Paranoid PD.
D. Passive-aggressive PD.
E. Schizoid PD.

The correct response is option A: BPD.

Compared with the general population, BPD and dependent PD are much more prevalent in the clinical population (Torgersen 2012; Torgersen et al. 2001). Other PDs somewhat more common in clinical populations include narcissistic, histrionic, avoidant, and schizotypal PDs. Schizoid PD is less common in clinical populations than in the general population (option E). Passive-aggressive (option D), paranoid (option C), antisocial, and obsessive-compulsive (option B) PDs are relatively weakly more common in the clinical population. Data suggest that it is not the degree of suffering that leads patients to seek clinical treatment but rather personality traits such as degree of extroversion and dependence. **(p. 115)**

6.5   What developmental trend is observed in Cluster B PDs compared with Cluster A PDs?

A. Persons with Cluster B PDs tend to be younger.
B. Persons with Cluster B PDs tend to be older.
C. Persons with Cluster B PDs tend to be middle-aged.
D. Persons with Cluster B PDs are just as likely to be any age.
E. Persons with Cluster A and B PDs tend to be similar ages.

The correct response is option A: Persons with Cluster B PDs tend to be younger.

Persons with borderline, antisocial, histrionic, and narcissistic (Cluster B) PDs seem to be younger, whereas those with schizoid and obsessive-compulsive PDs are older. These findings are in accordance with studies showing a strong developmental trend from Cluster B disorder to Cluster A and a somewhat weaker change to Cluster C disorders (Seivewright et al. 2002). The reason for the age differences in disorders may be that people become less impulsive and overtly aggressive as they age. Agreeableness and conscientiousness increase with age (Srivastava et al. 2003). Cluster B PDs are typically negatively correlated with agreeableness and conscientiousness (Saulsman and Page 2004). **(pp. 118–119)**

6.6   Although many PDs are related to lower education, which PD goes against this trend and seems to be correlated with higher education?

A. Histrionic PD.
B. Narcissistic PD.
C. Obsessive-compulsive PD.
D. Paranoid PD.
E. Schizoid PD.

The correct response is option C: Obsessive-compulsive PD.

Torgersen et al. (2001) observed that paranoid and avoidant PDs and traits and schizoid, schizotypal, antisocial, borderline, dependent, and self-defeating personality traits were related to lower education. In this study, histrionic, narcissistic, and passive-aggressive PDs were unrelated to education. Those with obsessive-compulsive PD or traits had higher education. Grant et al. (2004) found that lower income was related to all of the studied (Wave 1) personality disorders, except obsessive-compulsive PD. Lenzenweger et al. (2007) found that only BPD was related to unemployment. **(pp. 122)**

6.7   What is the relationship between quality of life and number of criteria fulfilled for any specific PD?

A. Quality of life decreases with increasing number of criteria fulfilled in a linear relationship.
B. Quality of life is associated with number of criteria fulfilled only to a limited extent.

C. Quality of life is equally affected beyond a certain number of fulfilled criteria.

D. Quality of life and number of criteria show a relationship in only certain PDs.

E. Quality of life is affected only after reaching a certain threshold of criteria fulfilled.

The correct response is option A: Quality of life decreases with increasing number of criteria fulfilled in a linear relationship.

For both quality of life and dysfunction, there is a perfect linear dose-response relationship to number of criteria fulfilled for all PDs (Torgersen et al. 2001). Thus, if a person has one criterion fulfilled for one or another PD (option D), the quality of life is lower and dysfunction is higher than among those with no criteria fulfilled (option B). Those with two criteria fulfilled for one or more specific disorders have lower quality of life than those patients meeting just one criterion and so on (option C). This result indicates that there are no arguments for any specific number of criteria to define a PD if one uses quality of life or dysfunction as validation variables. There is no natural cutoff point before or after which quality of life or dysfunction is not affected (option E). **(pp. 123–124)**

6.8   Which PD is associated with the highest levels of dysfunction and poorest quality of life?

A. Avoidant PD.

B. BPD.

C. Dependent PD.

D. Histrionic PD.

E. Obsessive-compulsive PD.

The correct response is option A: Avoidant PD.

All studies taken together show that reduced quality of life and dysfunction are highest among those with avoidant PD. Next come schizotypal PD and BPD, then follow paranoid, schizoid, dependent, and antisocial PDs. There are few studies showing impaired quality of life for histrionic, narcissistic, or obsessive-compulsive PDs. **(p. 125)**

6.9   Which of the following individuals is most likely to have a diagnosis of a PD?

A. A 25-year-old male medical student living with his wife in the suburbs.

B. A 26-year-old separated female with an associate's degree living in a rural area.

C. A 27-year-old female with a GED living with her partner on the outskirts of a city.

D. A 28-year-old divorced man without a high school degree living alone in a city.

E. A 29-year-old single woman working as an attorney in a metropolitan area.

The correct response is option D: A 28-year-old divorced man without a high school degree living alone in a city.

The highest prevalence of PDs in the general population is observed among subjects with lower education living in populated areas, for example, in a city center. They often have a history of divorce and separation and are more often living without a partner. It is typical for those with PDs (with the exception for those with obsessive-compulsive PD) to live alone. In some cases, they have never married (antisocial, dependent), have a history of frequent divorces (borderline), are divorced (paranoid), or are not married (histrionic) when interviewed. **(pp. 119–122)**

6.10   Which of the following PDs is more common in women?

A. Antisocial PD.
B. BPD.
C. Dependent PD.
D. Schizoid PD.
E. Schizotypal PD.

The correct response is option C: Dependent PD.

The most clear-cut results from research are that men tend to be antisocial, schizoid (options A, D), and narcissistic and that women tend to be histrionic and dependent. No clear gender bias for schizotypal PD is observed in the literature (option E). In patient samples, BPD is not more prevalent among women then among men (Alnæs and Torgersen 1988; Fossati et al. 2003; Golomb et al. 1995). In one study of patients, BPD was, in fact, more common among men (option B) than among women (Carter et al. 1999). **(p. 117)**

References

Alnæs R, Torgersen S: DSM-III symptom disorders (Axis I) and personality disorders (Axis II) in an outpatient population. Acta Psychiatr Scand 78:348–355, 1988 3195356
Carter JD, Joyce PR, Mulder RT, et al: Gender differences in the frequency of personality disorders in depressed outpatients. J Pers Disord 13:67–74, 1999 10228928
Durbin EC, Klein DN: Ten-year stability of personality disorders among outpatients with mood disorders. J Abnorm Psychol 115:75–84, 2006 16492098
Ferro T, Klein DN, Schwartz JE, et al: 30-month stability of personality disorder diagnoses in depressed outpatients. Am J Psychiatry 155:653–659, 1998 9585717
Fossati A, Feeney JA, Donati D, et al: Personality disorders and adult attachment dimensions in a mixed psychiatric sample: a multivariate study. J Nerv Ment Dis 191:30–37, 2003 12544597
Golomb M, Fava M, Abraham M, et al: Gender differences in personality disorders. Am J Psychiatry 152:579–582, 1995 7694907
Grant BF, Hasin DS, Stinson FR, et al: Prevalence, correlates, and disability of personality disorders in the United States: results from the national epidemiologic survey on alcohol and related conditions. J Clin Psychiatry 65:948–958, 2004 15291684
Grilo CM, Sanislow CA, Gunderson JG, et al: Two-year stability and change of schizotypal, borderline, avoidant, and obsessive-compulsive personality disorders. J Consult Clin Psychol 72:767–775, 2004 15482035
Johnson JG, Cohen P, Kasen S, et al: Cumulative prevalence of personality disorders between adolescence and adulthood. Acta Psychiar Scand 118:410–413, 2008 18644003
Lenzenweger MF, Lane MC, Loranger AW, et al: DSM-IV personality disorders in the national comorbidity survey replication. Biol Psychiatry 62:553–564, 2007 17217923

Saulsman LM, Page AC: The five-factor model and personality disorders empirical literature: a meta-analytic review. Clin Psychol Rev 23:1055–1085, 2004 14729423

Seivewright H, Tyrer P, Johnson T: Change in personality status in neurotic disorders. Lancet 359:2253–2254, 2002 12103293

Shea MT, Stout R, Gunderson J, et al: Short-term diagnostic stability of schizotypal, borderline, avoidant, and obsessive-compulsive personality disorders. Am J Psychiatry 159:2036–2041, 2002 12450953

Skodol AE, Gunderson JG, Shea MT, et al: The Collaborative Longitudinal Personality Disorders Study (CLPS): overview and implications. J Pers Disord 19:487–504, 2005 16274278

Srivastava S, John OP, Gosling SD, et al: Development of personality in early and middle adulthood: set like plaster or persistent change? J Pers Soc Psychol 84:1041–1053, 2003 12757147

Torgersen S: Epidemiology, in The Oxford Handbook of Personality Disorders. Edited by Widiger TA. Oxford, UK, Oxford University Press, 2012, pp 186–205

Torgersen S, Kringlen E, Cramer V: The prevalence of personality disorders in a community sample. Arch Gen Psychiatry 58:590–596, 2001 11386989

Zanarini MC, Frankenburg FR, Hennen J, et al: Prediction of the 10-year course of borderline personality disorder. Am J Psychiatry 163:827–832, 2006 16648323

CHAPTER 7

Manifestations, Assessment, and Differential Diagnosis

7.1 DSM-5 Section III provides diagnostic criteria for which of the following personality disorders (PDs)?

A. Dependent.
B. Histrionic.
C. Paranoid.
D. Schizoid.
E. Schizotypal.

The correct response is option E: Schizotypal.

DSM-5 Section III provides diagnostic criteria for 6 of the 10 Section II categories—antisocial, avoidant, borderline, narcissistic, obsessive-compulsive, and schizotypal—that are judged to have the most empirical evidence of validity and/or clinical utility. The other four Section II PDs (options A, B, C, D) and all other presentations that meet the Section III general criteria for a PD are diagnosed as personality disorder–trait specified (PD-TS) in the alternative model. **(p. 132)**

7.2 Criterion A of the general criteria for the diagnosis of PD in the alternative DSM-5 model of PD requires moderate or greater impairment in which of the following areas of personality functioning?

A. Conscientiousness.
B. Emotional stability.
C. Extraversion.
D. Lucidity.
E. Self/interpersonal relatedness.

The correct response is option E: Self/interpersonal relatedness.

The general diagnostic criteria for a PD in Section II of DSM-5 indicate that a pattern of inner experience and behavior is manifest by characteristic patterns of 1) cognition (i.e., ways of perceiving and interpreting self, other people, and events); 2) affectivity (i.e., the range, intensity, lability, and appropriateness of emotional response); 3) interpersonal functioning; and 4) impulse control. Persons with PDs are expected to have manifestations in at least two of these areas. In contrast, the Section III general criteria focus on impairment in personality functioning and the presence of pathological personality traits. Personality functioning consists of sense of self (identity and self-direction) and interpersonal relatedness (empathy and intimacy), capturing aspects of all four Section II areas. Options A–D are considered to be personality trait domains whose polar opposites are considered to be pathological personality trait domains. For example, Conscientiousness (vs. Disinhibition), Emotional Stability (vs. Negative Affectivity), Extraversion (vs. Detachment), and Lucidity (vs. Psychoticism). **(p. 134)**

7.3   Which one of the following is one of the five broad pathological personality trait domains in DSM-5 Section III?

   A. Detachment.
   B. Submissiveness.
   C. Impulsivity.
   D. Manipulativeness.
   E. Eccentricity.

   The correct response is option A: Detachment.

   Pathological personality traits in DSM-5 Section III are organized into five broad domains: Negative Affectivity, Detachment, Antagonism, Disinhibition, and Psychoticism. Within these five broad *trait domains* are 25 specific *trait facets* that have been developed initially from a review of existing trait models and then through iterative research on samples of persons who sought mental health services. Options B–E are specific trait facets within the remaining four broad pathological personality domains. Submissiveness is a facet of Negative Affectivity. Impulsivity is facet of Disinhibition, Manipulativeness is a facet of Antagonism, and Eccentricity is a facet of Psychoticism. **(pp. 135–136)**

7.4   In DSM-5 Section III, alternative diagnostic model of PDs, the Level of Personality Functioning Scale (LPFS) assesses which of the following areas of personality and adaptive functioning?

   A. Agreeableness.
   B. Conscientiousness.
   C. Empathy.
   D. Extroversion.
   E. Openness.

The correct response is option C: Empathy.

Disturbances in *self-functioning* and *interpersonal functioning* constitute the core of personality psychopathology. In the alternative Section III diagnostic model, they are evaluated on a continuum, using the LPFS. The LPFS assesses capacities that lie at the heart of personality and adaptive functioning. Self-functioning involves identity and self-direction; interpersonal functioning involves empathy and intimacy.

Identity is defined as the experience of oneself as unique, with clear boundaries between self and others; stability of self-esteem and accuracy of self-appraisal; and the capacity for, and ability to regulate, a range of emotional experience. *Self-direction* is the pursuit of coherent and meaningful short-term and life goals; the utilization of constructive and prosocial internal standards of behavior; and the ability to self-reflect productively. *Empathy* is the comprehension and appreciation of others' experiences and motivations; tolerance of differing perspectives; and an understanding of the effects of one's own behavior on others. *Intimacy* reflects the depth and duration of connection with others; a desire and capacity for closeness; and a mutuality of regard reflected in interpersonal behavior. The LPFS utilizes each of these elements to differentiate five levels of impairment, ranging from *little or no impairment* (i.e., healthy, adaptive functioning; Level 0), to *some* (Level 1), *moderate* (Level 2), *severe* (Level 3), and *extreme* (Level 4) impairment. The other options given are among the five-factor personality traits. **(p. 135)**

7.5   Which of the following PDs is least likely to have impairment in the domains of social, work, and leisure?

A. Avoidant.
B. Borderline.
C. Obsessive-compulsive.
D. Schizotypal.

The correct response is option C: Obsessive-compulsive.

When patients with different PDs were compared with each other on levels of functional impairment, those with severe PDs such as borderline PD (BPD) and schizotypal PD (options B, D) were found to have significantly more impairment at work, in social relationships, and at leisure than patients with less severe PDs, such as obsessive-compulsive PD (OCPD). Patients with avoidant PD (option A) had intermediate levels of impairment. Even the less impaired patients with PDs (e.g., OCPD), however, had moderate to severe impairment in at least one area of functioning (or a Global Assessment of Functioning rating of 60 or less; Skodol et al. 2002). **(p. 144)**

7.6   Agreement between the patient and an informant about personality traits and interpersonal problems is highest for which of the following PDs?

A. Avoidant.
B. Borderline.
C. Dependent.
D. Narcissistic.
E. Paranoid.

The correct response is option B: Borderline.

Agreement between patient and informant on pathological personality traits, temperament, and interpersonal problems appears to be somewhat better than on the actual diagnosis of DSM PDs. Informants usually report more personality psychopathology than patients. Agreement on PDs between patient self-assessments and informant assessments is highest for Cluster B disorders (borderline, excluding narcissistic PD), lower for clusters A (paranoid) (option E) and C (avoidant, dependent) (options A, C), and lowest for traits related to narcissism (option D) and entitlement, as might be expected. **(pp. 146–147)**

7.7   Which is the only PD that cannot be diagnosed before age 18 years?

A. Antisocial.
B. Avoidant.
C. Borderline.
D. Dependent.
E. Schizotypal.

The correct response is option A: Antisocial.

Antisocial PD is the only diagnosis not given before age 18 years; an adolescent exhibiting significant antisocial behavior before age 18 is diagnosed with conduct disorder. DSM-5 states, however, that some manifestations of PD are usually recognizable by adolescence or earlier and that PDs can be diagnosed in persons younger than age 18 years who have manifested symptoms for at least 1 year. **(p. 148)**

7.8   Which PD may become more pronounced with age?

A. Antisocial.
B. Avoidant.
C. Paranoid.
D. Dependent.
E. Schizotypal.

The correct response is option E: Schizotypal.

Regarding the course of a PD, DSM-5 states that PDs are relatively stable over time (options B, D), although certain of them (e.g., antisocial PD and BPD) may become somewhat attenuated with age (options A, C), whereas others (e.g., obsessive-compulsive PD and schizotypal PD) may not or may, in fact, become more pronounced. Also the degree of stability may not necessarily pertain to all of the features of all DSM-5 PDs equally. **(p. 148)**

7.9 The externalizing "meta-cluster" of disorders is characterized primarily by which of the following personality traits?

A. Detachment.
B. Disinhibition.
C. Extraversion.
D. Negative affectivity.
E. Psychoticism.

The correct response is option B: Disinhibition.

Externalizing disorders, such as conduct disorder, substance-related and addictive disorders, and antisocial PD are characterized primarily by Disinhibition, that is, an "orientation toward immediate gratification, leading to impulsive behavior, driven by current thoughts, feelings, and external stimuli, without regard for past learning or future consequences" (American Psychiatric Association 2013, p. 780). These individuals may also be characterized by Antagonism.

Internalizing disorders, such as anxiety and depressive disorders and avoidant PD, are characterized by Negative Affectivity (option D), that is, "frequent and intense experiences of high levels of a wide range of negative emotions (e.g., anxiety, depression, guilt/shame, worry, anger) and their behavioral (e.g., self-harm) and interpersonal (e.g., dependency) manifestations" (American Psychiatric Association 2013, p. 779). BPD straddles both spectra. Detachment (option A) and Psychoticism (option E) are not primarily seen in either the externalizing or internalizing disorders and are likely seen in other personality disorders such as OCPD (Detachment) and schizotypal (Detachment and Psychoticism). Extraversion (option C) is the polar opposite of Detachment and is not considered a pathological personality trait. **(pp. 153–154)**

7.10 As part of the assessment in the outpatient psychiatric clinic, a patient is administered the Personality Inventory for DSM-5 (PID-5). The patient scores high on the PID-5 on traits of negative affectivity, antagonism, and disinhibition. On the basis of these findings, which of the PDs is the most likely diagnosis for this patient?

A. Antisocial.
B. Avoidant.
C. Borderline.
D. Narcissistic.
E. Schizotypal.

The correct response is option C: Borderline.

Individual PDs in Section III are characterized by different combinations of underlying trait domains: antisocial PD (option A) is a combination of Antagonism and Disinhibition; BPD is a combination of Negative Affectivity, Antagonism, and Disinhibition; avoidant PD (option B) is a combination of Negative Affectivity and Detachment; schizotypal PD (option E) is a combination of Psychoticism and Detachment; and obsessive-compulsive PD is a combination of Conscientiousness (the opposite of Disinhibition), Negative Affectivity, and Detachment. Of the specific PDs in Section III, only narcissistic PD (option D) is characterized by a single trait domain (Antagonism). The personality trait model is operationalized by use of the PID-5, which can be completed in its self-report form by patients. **(pp. 136, 154)**

References

American Psychiatric Association: Diagnostic and Statistical Manual of Mental Disorders, 5th Edition. Washington, DC, American Psychiatric Association, 2013

Skodol AE, Gunderson JG, McGlashan TH, et al: Functional impairment in patients with schizotypal, borderline, avoidant, or obsessive-compulsive personality disorder. Am J Psychiatry 159:276–283, 2002 11823271

CHAPTER 8

Course and Outcome

8.1   Which of the following is a key concept of personality disorders (PDs) in both the DSM-5 and the ICD-10?

A. Classification of categories.
B. Definitions of traits.
C. Criteria for diagnosis.
D. Stability over time.
E. Impact on function.

The correct response is option D: Stability over time.

Although the concept of stability is salient in both of the major classification systems, DSM-5 (American Psychiatric Association 2013) and ICD-10 (World Health Organization 1992), the two systems differ somewhat in their classification and definitions and criteria for diagnosis and impact of PD on functioning (options A, B, C, E), and thus they demonstrate only moderate convergence for some diagnoses (Ottosson et al. 2002). **(p. 165)**

8.2   According to Carpenter and Gunderson, the impairment in functioning observed for borderline PD (BPD) over a 5-year period was comparable to the impairment of functioning in patients with which of the following disorders?

A. Major depression.
B. Bipolar disorder.
C. Panic disorder.
D. Social phobia.
E. Schizophrenia.

The correct response is option E: Schizophrenia.

Carpenter and Gunderson (1977) reported that the impairment in functioning observed for BPD was comparable to that observed for patients with schizophrenia over a 5-year period. **(p. 166)**

8.3   What was the intent in DSM-III to place the PDs on a separate axis (Axis II) of the multiaxial system?

   A. Assess for presence of disorders often overlooked in the presence of an Axis I disorder.
   B. Diagnostic construct of PD did not evolve over time.
   C. Recognize the instability of both Axis I and Axis II PDs.
   D. Encourage clinicians to focus on a specific disorder.
   E. Recognize the pattern of instability of personality traits.

The correct response is option A: Assess for presence of disorders often overlooked in the presence of an Axis I disorder.

The DSM-III indicates that the assignment to Axis II was intended, in part, to encourage clinicians to assess for additional disorders that might be overlooked when focusing on Axis I psychiatric disorders. Conceptually, this reflected, in part, the putative stability of PDs relative to the episodically unstable course of so-called Axis I psychiatric disorders (Grilo et al. 1998; Shea and Yen 2003; Skodol 1997; Skodol et al. 2002) (options C, D, E). The diagnostic construct of PD has evolved considerably over the past few decades, and substantial changes have occurred over time in the number and types of specific PD diagnoses and their criteria (option B). **(pp. 165–166)**

8.4   The placement of PDs on a separate axis facilitated which of the following research issues?

   A. Increased research focus on Axis I disorders.
   B. Development and utilization of structured and standardized clinical interviewing.
   C. Recognition of the effect of Axis I disorders on PDs.
   D. Increased accuracy of diagnosis of the different PDs.
   E. Increased accuracy of diagnosis of Axis I disorders.

The correct response is option B: Development and utilization of structured and standardized clinical interviewing.

The separation of PDs to Axis II in DSM-III (American Psychiatric Association 1980) contributed to increased research attention on PDs separate from Axis I disorders (option A) (Blashfield and McElroy 1987). The development and utilization of a number of structured and standardized approaches to clinical interviewing and diagnosis during the 1980s represented notable advances, which were reflective of the greater attention given to PDs as they were separated onto Axis II (Zimmerman 1994). Options C, D, and E are incorrect because they are not related to the PDs being separated onto Axis II. **(pp. 166–167)**

8.5   Research regarding the long-term course of PDs involves the repeated-measures approach (test-retest), which may address the problem of "regression to the mean." What is an untoward effect on the reliability of study data caused by this methodology?

A. Participants systematically report or endorse fewer problems on repeat interview by reporting fewer symptoms.
B. Participants prefer to remain in one study for an extended duration.
C. Participants will have a tendency to underreport symptoms at baseline.
D. Participants tend to report more symptoms on repeat interview to increase interview times.
E. Participants become more consistent on repeat interview over an extended period of time.

The correct response is option A: Participants systematically report or endorse fewer problems on repeat interview by reporting fewer symptoms.

Test-retest reliability is relevant for addressing, in part, the well-known problem of "regression to the mean" in repeated-measures studies (Nesselroade et al. 1980). It has been argued that the multiwave or repeated-measures approach lessens the effects of regression to the mean (Lenzenweger 1999). This might be the case in terms of the obvious decreases in severity with time. Participants may eventually leave a study for an extended duration (option B). Very symptomatic participants meeting eligibility at study entry are likely to show some improvement because by definition they are already reporting high levels of symptoms at baseline rather than underreporting symptoms at baseline (option C). However, other effects need to be considered whenever assessments are repeated within a study. Shea and Yen (2003) noted that repeated-measures studies of both PD (Loranger et al. 1991) and other mental disorder (Robins 1985) diagnoses have found hints that participants systematically report or endorse fewer problems during repeat interviews to reduce interview time (option D). Multiple incentives for overreporting (e.g., admission to a desirable treatment facility) and underreporting (e.g., discharge from a hospital) can be present throughout the duration of a study (option E). **(p. 169)**

8.6   If diagnosed during adolescence, which of the following diagnoses predicts substantially elevated risk for antisocial behavior during adulthood?

A. Attention-deficit/hyperactivity disorder.
B. Bipolar disorder.
C. Conduct disorder.
D. Obsessive-compulsive disorder.
E. Social phobia.

The correct response is option C: Conduct disorder.

The diagnosis of conduct disorder during adolescence is required for the diagnosis of antisocial PD to be given to adults. This definitional isomorphism is one likely reason for the consistently strong associations between conduct disorder and later antisocial PD in the literature. This is, however, more than an artifactual relationship, because longitudinal research has documented that children and adolescents with early-onset behavior disorders have substantially elevated risk for antisocial behavior during adulthood (Moffitt 1993; Robins 1966). **(p. 170)**

8.7   Why is determining early onset of PDs in adolescence difficult?

A. Consistency of personality traits decreases with age.
B. Consistency of personality traits is highest during adolescence.
C. Adolescents are unreliable in their self-report to the structured interviews.
D. Adolescence is a period of profound changes and flux in personality and identity.
E. The effect of peer pressure during adolescence confounds the presentation of personality traits.

The correct response is option D: Adolescence is a period of profound changes and flux in personality and identity.

Determining early onset of PDs is impossible because adolescence is a period of profound changes and flux in personality and identity. A critical review of the longitudinal literature on personality traits throughout the lifespan revealed that personality traits are less stable during childhood and adolescence than they are later in life (Roberts and DelVecchio 2000) (option A). Consistency of personality traits is highest in adulthood (50+ years of age) (option B). Options C and E are incorrect because they are not supported by research findings. **(p. 171)**

8.8   The temperamental feature of being withdrawn in childhood is noted to be a precursor of which of the following PDs in adulthood?

A. Avoidant.
B. Borderline.
C. Dependent.
D. Paranoid.
E. Schizotypal.

The correct response is option E: Schizotypal.

Studies have noted early odd and withdrawn patterns preceding schizotypal PD in adults (Wolff et al. 1991). **(p. 171)**

8.9   Which of the following PD clusters tends to show significant improvement with age?

A. Cluster A.
B. Cluster B.
C. Cluster C.

The correct response is option B: Cluster B.

Seivewright et al. (2002) reported that Cluster B PD diagnoses (antisocial, histrionic) showed significant improvements, whereas Cluster A (schizoid, schizotypal, paranoid) and Cluster C (obsessional, avoidant) appeared to worsen with age. The Seivewright et al. (2002) findings, however, are limited by the two-point cross-sectional assessment, which could not address the nature of changes during the intervening period. **(p. 172)**

8.10 Which of the following PDs is associated with a significantly longer duration of time to achieve remission (defined as good social and vocational functioning in addition to minimal PD symptoms) than all other PDs?

A. Avoidant.
B. Histrionic.
C. Borderline.
D. Paranoid.
E. Schizoid.

The correct response is option C: Borderline.

In their report of 16 years of prospective follow-up, Zanarini et al. (2012) showed that patients with BPD were significantly slower to achieve remission (defined in the McLean Study of Adult Development as good social and vocational functioning, in addition to minimal PD symptoms) than the comparison group with other PDs. **(p. 178)**

8.11 What did the 10 years of prospective yearly multimethod follow-up in the Collaborative Longitudinal Personality Disorders Study (CLPS) demonstrate about the course of BPD?

A. High rates of diagnostic remission and low rates of relapse (return to diagnostic threshold), but severe and enduring social functioning impairment.
B. Low rates of diagnostic remission and low rates of relapse (return to diagnostic threshold), but severe and enduring social functioning impairment.
C. High rates of diagnostic remission and high rates of relapse (return to diagnostic threshold), but severe and enduring social functioning impairment.
D. Low rates of diagnostic remission and high rates of relapse (return to diagnostic threshold), but severe and enduring social functioning impairment.
E. High rates of diagnostic remission, low rates of relapse (return to diagnostic threshold), and decreased social functioning impairment.

The correct response is option A: High rates of diagnostic remission and low rates of relapse (return to diagnostic threshold), but severe and enduring social functioning impairment.

These findings—based on 10 years of prospective yearly multimethod follow-up—indicate that the course of BPD is characterized by high rates of diagnostic remission and low rates of relapse (return to diagnostic threshold), but severe and enduring social functioning impairment (Gunderson et al. 2011). **(p. 175)**

References

American Psychiatric Association: Diagnostic and Statistical Manual of Mental Disorders, 3rd Edition. Washington, DC, American Psychiatric Association, 1980

American Psychiatric Association: Diagnostic and Statistical Manual of Mental Disorders, 5th Edition. Washington, DC, American Psychiatric Association, 2013

Blashfield RK, McElroy RA: The 1985 journal literature on the personality disorders. Compr Psychiatry 28:536–546, 1987 3319384

Carpenter WT, Gunderson JG: Five-year follow-up comparison of borderline and schizophrenic patients. Compr Psychiatry 18:567–571, 1977 923229

Grilo CM, McGlashan TH, Oldham JM: Course and stability of personality disorders. J Pract Psychiatry Behav Health 4:61–75, 1998

Gunderson JG, Stout RL, McGlashan TH, et al: Ten-year course of borderline personality disorder: psychopathology and function from the Collaborative Longitudinal Personality Disorders Study. Arch Gen Psychiatry 68:827–837, 2011 21464343

Lenzenweger MF: Stability and change in personality disorder features: the longitudinal study of personality disorders. Arch Gen Psychiatry 56:1009–1015, 1999 10565501

Loranger AW, Lenzenweger MF, Gartner AF, et al: Trait-state artifacts and the diagnosis of personality disorders. Arch Gen Psychiatry 48:720–728, 1991 1883255

Moffitt TE: Adolescence-limited and life-course-persistent antisocial behavior: a developmental taxonomy. Psychol Rev 100:674–701, 1993 8255953

Nesselroade JR, Stigler SM, Baltes PB: Regression toward the mean and the study of change. Psychol Bull 88:622–637, 1980

Ottosson H, Ekselius L, Grann M, et al: Cross-system concordance of personality disorder diagnoses of DSM-IV and diagnostic criteria for research of ICD-10. J Pers Disord 16:283–292, 2002 12136684

Roberts BW, DelVecchio WF: The rank-order consistency of personality traits from childhood to old age: a quantitative review of longitudinal studies. Psychol Bull 126:3–25, 2000 10668348

Robins LN: Deviant children grown up: a sociological and psychiatric study of sociopathic personality. Baltimore, MD, Williams & Wilkins, 1966

Robins LN: Epidemiology: reflections on testing the validity of psychiatric interviews. Arch Gen Psychiatry 42:918–924, 1985 3899050

Seivewright H, Tyrer P, Johnson T: Change in personality status in neurotic disorders. Lancet 359:2253–2254, 2002 12103293

Shea MT, Yen S: Stability as a distinction between axis I and axis II disorders. J Pers Disord 17:373–386, 2003 14632373

Skodol AE: Classification, assessment, and differential diagnosis of personality disorders. J Pract Psychiatry Behav Health 3:261–274, 1997

Skodol AE, Siever LJ, Livesley WJ, et al: The borderline diagnosis II: biology, genetics, and clinical course. Biol Psychiatry 15:951–963, 2002

Wolff S, Townshend R, McGuire RJ, et al: Schizoid personality in childhood and adult life, II: adult adjustment and the continuity with schizotypal personality disorder. Br J Psychiatry 159:620–629, 1991 1756337

World Health Organization: International Statistical Classification of Diseases and Related Health Problems, 10th Revision. Geneva, World Health Organization, 1992

Zanarini MC, Frankenburg FR, Reich DB, et al: Attainment and stability of sustained symptomatic remission and recovery among patients with borderline personality disorder and axis II comparison subjects: a 16-year prospective follow-up study. Am J Psychiatry 169:476–483, 2012 22737693

Zimmerman M: Diagnosing personality disorders. A review of issues and research methods. Arch Gen Psychiatry 51:225–245, 1994 8122959

CHAPTER 9

Therapeutic Alliance

9.1 In research on the treatment of personality disorders (PDs), which of the following is the most robust predictor of treatment outcome?

A. Therapeutic alliance.
B. Duration of therapy.
C. Therapeutic modality.
D. Socioeconomic factors.
E. Self-harm history.

The correct response is option A: Therapeutic alliance.

It is sometimes difficult to determine a priori who will benefit from what treatment with whom, but one factor—therapeutic alliance—has stood out in the research literature as the most robust predictor of outcome (Horvath et al. 2011; Safran et al. 2011). There are a number of evidence-based, effective brief therapies, so duration of therapy (option B) would not be the most robust predictor of treatment outcome. Additionally, there are a variety of therapeutic modalities (option C) with a strong evidence base of efficacy. Socioeconomic factors (option D) and self-harm history (option E), while important to address in therapy, do not preclude a beneficial treatment outcome. **(p. 189)**

9.2 The concept of therapeutic alliance is attributed originally to which of the following people?

A. Gerald Adler.
B. Heinz Kohut.
C. Otto Kernberg.
D. Sigmund Freud.
E. Donald Winnicott.

The correct response is option D: Sigmund Freud.

The concept of the therapeutic alliance is often traced back to Freud, who observed very early in his work the need to convey interest in and sympathy to the patient to engage him or her in a collaborative treatment endeavor (Meissner 1996; Safran and Muran 2000). Freud (1912/1958) also delineated an aspect of the transference—the unobjectionable positive transference—which is an attachment that should not be analyzed because it serves as the motivation for the patient to collaborate. This was an early precursor to the modern empirical evidence showing that alliance is related to treatment outcome across modalities. **(p. 190)**

9.3 A patient who has had a good therapeutic alliance with his psychiatrist for a year suddenly appears dissatisfied with the treatment during a session. He calls later and leaves a message wanting to discontinue therapy. Which of the following is the recommended therapist response?

A. Transfer the patient to the care of another psychiatrist.
B. Suggest the patient return to share his concerns.
C. Refer the patient to the state medical board complaints office.
D. Contact a lawyer for medicolegal advice.
E. Discuss the case with another psychiatrist to review therapist counter-transference.

The correct response is option B: Suggest the patient return to share his concerns.

Skilled therapists and supervisors are aware that ruptures and threats to a therapeutic alliance are common and to be expected in treatment, especially with patients with PDs. These ruptures may offer excellent opportunities to engage the patient in a collaborative effort to observe and learn about that patient's own style. Addressing and working through threats to the therapeutic alliance can be excellent opportunities for clinical improvement. Evidence has shown that strains or ruptures in the alliance are often related to unilateral termination (Safran et al. 2011). Asking this patient to come in and discuss his wish to terminate is the correct response because it is the only response that brings the patient and therapist together to provide the opportunity to negotiate a rupture in the therapeutic alliance, which, if skillfully addressed, can strengthen the alliance, leading to a better outcome. None of the other responses bring the patient and therapist together (Safran et al. 2011; Strauss et al. 2006). **(pp. 191–192)**

9.4 Which of the following is a characteristic clinical challenge when treating a patient with a Cluster A (paranoid/schizoid/schizotypal) PD?

A. Establishing a working alliance with the patient.
B. Unstable emotional and cognitive states of the patient.
C. Patient sensitivity to treatment recommendations as criticism.
D. Patient's need for control of the treatment process.
E. Addressing patient's demandingness.

The correct response is option A: Establishing a working alliance with the patient.

Patients with Cluster A PDs often mistrust or do not want close interpersonal relationships. They have pronounced paranoid or alienated features making development of a therapeutic alliance difficult (Lingiardi et al. 2005). Unstable emotional and cognitive states (option B) and demandingness (option E) are characteristic of Cluster B PDs. Sensitivity to criticism and need for control (options C, D) are features that are characteristic of Cluster C PDs. **(pp. 193–205)**

9.5   A patient who starts therapy with a new psychiatrist is very complimentary at the first appointment. By the third appointment, the patient voices numerous verbal criticisms and expresses anger with the clinical treatment. There are no inappropriate threats or concerns to the psychiatrist's safety, and the patient makes another appointment. Which of the following is the most helpful response the psychiatrist could employ for this patient?

A. Terminate therapy and discharge the patient.
B. Contact a malpractice lawyer for advice.
C. Interpret the reason for the anger.
D. Tolerate the expression of anger.
E. Identify and explain the development of transference.

The correct response is option D: Tolerate the expression of anger.

Although it is important to distinguish anger from a therapeutic alliance rupture, it is helpful when the therapist can tolerate the patient's expression of anger and aggression early in treatment, provided there is no concern about transgressing limits or a safety boundary. Until a therapeutic alliance has been developed, reflection, interpretation, and transference identification can challenge and distress the patient and threaten the alliance (options C, E). Terminating therapy (option A) and contacting a malpractice lawyer (option B) would be premature and could sever any alliance. **(pp. 201–202)**

9.6   Which of the following is the appropriate therapeutic stance in the early stages of treatment with a patient who has narcissistic PD?

A. Tolerate the patient's grandiosity.
B. Agree with the patient's sense of self-importance.
C. Firmly establish and demonstrate therapist control.
D. Use numerous early interpretations.
E.   Ask for proof of grandiose claims.

The correct response is option A: Tolerate the patient's grandiosity.

The therapist must tolerate the patient's narcissistic grandiosity and vulnerability in the early stages of treatment without having to agree with (option B) or challenge it (options C, D, E) until a later time when a therapeutic alliance is developed. **(pp. 202–203)**

9.7 With respect to the his or her therapeutic alliance, which of the following is characteristic of a person with Cluster C PDs during treatment?

A. Feels guilt and takes blame for situations with the therapist.
B. Develops a quick and deep alliance with the therapist.
C. Frequently alternates between idealizing and devaluing the therapist.
D. Has difficulty trusting the therapist.
E. Exploits and uses the therapist to gratify personal needs.

The correct response is option A: Feels guilt and takes blame for situations with the therapist.

Patients with Cluster C PDs frequently feel very guilty and internalize blame for situations even when there is none. Developing a quick and deep alliance, alternating between extremes of idealization and devaluation, and exploitation (options B, C, E) are characteristics of Cluster B PDs. Difficulty trusting the therapist (option D) is characteristic of Cluster A PDs (Stone 1993). **(p. 203)**

9.8 When providing therapy to a person with borderline PD (BPD), which of the following approaches carries the greatest risk of rupturing the therapeutic alliance?

A. Supportive psychotherapy.
B. Cognitive-behavioral therapy.
C. Psychoeducation.
D. Medication management.
E. Transference interpretations.

The correct response is option E: Transference interpretations.

The most challenging therapist intervention is making a transference interpretation, because examination of transference most intensely challenges the patient's personality difficulties. Supportive therapy, cognitive-behavioral therapy, psychoeducation, and medication management (options A, B, C, D) are typically less emotionally intense compared with the examination of transference issues (Bond et al. 1998). **(pp. 208–209)**

9.9 What is the recommended physician stance when prescribing medication to patients with PDs?

A. Directive expert.
B. Collaborative participant.
C. Passive responder.
D. Authoritarian leader.
E. Interpretive reflector.

The correct response is option B: Collaborative participant.

Gutheil (1982) suggested that there is a particular aspect of the therapeutic alliance—what he calls the *pharmacotherapeutic alliance*—that is relevant to the prescription of medications. In this formulation of the alliance, it is recommended that the physician adopt the stance of *participant prescribing*—that is, rather than adopting an authoritarian role, the clinician should make every effort to involve the patient as a collaborator who engages actively in goal setting and observing and evaluating the experience of using specific medications. The other options risk rupturing the therapeutic alliance in patients with PDs, who may, on the one hand, feel slighted if not prescribed medications (options C, E), as if their problems were not taken seriously, or, on the other hand, may perceive a prescription as the physician trying to "put something over" on them (options A, D). **(p. 211)**

9.10 During the inpatient hospitalization of a patient with BPD, a treatment team encounters escalating conflict with each other about the treatment. Which of the following is the recommended action?

A. Transfer the patient to a different unit.
B. Change the attending psychiatrist.
C. Have team members independently assess the patient and contribute opinions.
D. Request a second opinion to decide on treatment.
E. Hold a team meeting to communicate and have a common united approach.

The correct response is option E: Hold a team meeting to communicate and have a common united approach.

Conflict between team members as a result of splitting by the patient is common among inpatient teams when treating BPD. Skilled teams will recognize the development of splitting and meet regularly to communicate and to configure a common united treatment approach. The central consideration regarding the alliance in this treatment context is that there is always a team of individuals responsible for the patient. With patients with borderline issues, splitting tendencies frequently are quite pronounced. That means that communication and close collaboration among the members of a team are vital during every phase of the hospital treatment. Options A, B, C, and D would not address the underlying PD pathology and could reinforce the splitting behavior. **(pp. 211–212)**

References

Bond M, Banon E, Grenier M: Differential effects of interventions on the therapeutic alliance with patients with personality disorders. J Psychother Pract Res 7:301–318, 1998 9752641

Freud S: The dynamics of transference (1912), in The Standard Edition of the Complete Psychological Works of Sigmund Freud, Vol 12. Translated and edited by Strachey J. London, Hogarth Press, 1958, pp 99–108

Gutheil TG: The psychology of psychopharmacology. Bull Menninger Clin 46:321–330, 1982 7139146

Horvath AO, Del Re AC, Flukiger C, et al: Alliance in individual psychotherapy. Psychotherapy (Chic) 48:9–16, 2011 21401269

Lingiardi V, Filippucci L, Baiocco R: Therapeutic alliance evaluation in personality disorders psychotherapy. Psychother Res 15:45–53, 2005

Meissner WW: The Therapeutic Alliance. New Haven, CT, Yale University Press, 1996

Safran JD, Muran JC: Negotiating the Therapeutic Alliance. New York, Guilford, 2000

Safran JD, Muran JC, Eubanks-Carter C: Repairing alliance ruptures. Psychotherapy (Chic) 48:80–87, 2011 21401278

Stone MH: Abnormalities of Personality. New York, WW Norton, 1993

Strauss JL, Hayes AM, Johnson SL, et al: Early alliance, alliance ruptures, and symptom change in a nonrandomized trial of cognitive therapy for avoidant and obsessive-compulsive personality disorders. J Consult Clin Psychol 74:337–345, 2006 16649878

CHAPTER 10

Psychodynamic Psychotherapies and Psychoanalysis

10.1 Which of the following best describes the criteria for a diagnosis of borderline personality organization?

A. The patient's personality organization is characterized by primitive defense mechanisms, identity diffusion, and generally intact but unstable reality testing.
B. The patient's personality is characterized by primitive defense mechanisms, identity diffusion, and loss of reality testing.
C. The patient's personality organization is characterized by primitive defense mechanisms, an overly consolidated identity, and generally intact but unstable reality testing.
D. The patient's personality organization is characterized by primitive defense mechanisms, identity diffusion, and the patient meets DSM criteria for borderline personality disorder (BPD).
E. The patient's personality organization is characterized by primitive defense mechanisms and the patient meets criteria for any of the personality disorders (PDs) described in the DSM.

The correct response is option A: The patient's personality organization is characterized by primitive defense mechanisms, identity diffusion, and generally intact but unstable reality testing.

The three central features of borderline personality organization are the use of primitive defenses, identity diffusion, and generally intact but unstable reality testing. Psychotic patients, rather than patients with borderline personality organization, have a loss of reality testing (option B). Borderline personality organization is characterized by identity diffusion, which means that identity is insufficiently consolidated, rather than overly consolidated (option C). No DSM diagnosis is required to make the psychoanalytic diagnosis of borderline personality organization (options D, E). **(p. 223)**

10.2 Which of the following psychological mechanisms are most central to a psychoanalytic understanding of severe PDs?

A. Repression and reaction formation.
B. Splitting and projective identification.
C. Humor and sublimation.
D. A neurotic level of personality organization.
E. Significant absence of reality testing.

The correct response is option B: Splitting and projective identification.

Primitive defense mechanisms are central features of severe PDs. These primitive defense mechanisms include splitting and projective identification, along with idealization/devaluation, primitive denial, and omnipotent control. Repression and reaction formation (option A) are neurotic defenses, whereas humor and sublimation (option C) are mature defense mechanisms. Dominance of these neurotic and mature defense mechanisms characterizes neurotic and normal levels of personality organization (option D). Patients with severe PDs generally do not have significant absence of reality testing (option E). **(pp. 221–222)**

10.3 Which of the following is true of specific psychoanalytic schools of thought as they relate to PDs?

A. In conceptualizing PDs, self psychology places special emphasis on the importance of psychological conflicts.
B. In conceptualizing PDs, ego psychology places more emphasis than other schools on the role of deficient child rearing in giving rise to PDs.
C. In conceptualizing PDs, object relations theory focuses on the importance of mental representations of self and others.
D. In conceptualizing PDs, the relational and interpersonal schools of psychoanalysis understand pathological traits in terms of the interpersonal expression of inner aggressive drives.
E. In conceptualizing personality pathology, mentalization-based therapy (MBT) focuses on how inherited difficulties with mentalization, rather than childhood trauma, give rise to pathological character traits.

The correct response is option C: In conceptualizing PDs, object relations theory focuses on the importance of mental representations of self and others.

The central focus of object relations theory is mental representations of self and others. An emphasis on the nature of psychological conflict is central to the explanations of psychopathology offered by ego psychology (option A). Self psychology emphasizes lasting effects of early deficiencies in child rearing in the development of psychopathology (option B). The relational and interpersonal schools also focus on the importance of the relationship between the patient and the therapist and consider that the personality of both patient and therapist contribute to the experience that needs to be analyzed in the therapy (option D). MBT grows out of the attachment theory school of thought, which also focuses on mental representations that are formed through repeated interactions with attachment figures (option E). **(pp. 221–227)**

10.4   Which of the following is true regarding the appropriateness of psychoanalytic treatment for patients with PDs?

A. Psychoanalysis is not an effective treatment for PDs, and patients should be referred for treatment with other modalities.
B. Psychoanalysis is effective for patients with less severe PDs and requires no modifications for patients with more severe PDs.
C. Psychoanalysis may be an effective treatment for some patients without PDs but is rarely useful for patients with PDs.
D. Psychoanalysis has become a viable alternative for working with severe PDs as appropriate technical modifications have been developed and tested.
E. Psychoanalysis should never be a first-line treatment for any patients with a PD.

The correct response is option D: Psychoanalysis has become a viable alternative for working with severe PDs as appropriate technical modifications have been developed and tested.

Psychoanalysis developed around the treatment of "neurotic" disorders but evolved to focus on character pathology and PDs (option C). Currently, patients with higher-level PDs may be referred for psychoanalysis or forms of psychodynamic psychotherapy (options A, E). Psychoanalytic training and research is increasingly including technical modifications for working with lower-level PDs as well, and it is important to refer more disturbed patients to clinicians who have this training (option B). **(p. 236)**

10.5   Which of the following modalities of psychotherapy for PDs involves a combination of group sessions and individual sessions; focuses on the patient's capacity to reflect on and appreciate intentions, feelings, and motivations in self and others; and, in later stages of treatment, works toward achieving such reflective functioning in the patient-therapist interaction?

A. Transference-focused psychotherapy (TFP).
B. Supportive-expressive therapy.
C. Dialectical behavioral therapy (DBT).
D. Psychoanalysis.
E. MBT.

The correct response is option E: MBT.

MBT, rooted in attachment theory and in psychoanalysis, has been developed for Cluster B PDs; it was initially practiced as a day hospital treatment and generally combines individual sessions with group sessions. The technique centers on identifying moments when mentalization is lost. The therapist rewinds to the moment before the break, focusing on the momentary affects between patient and therapist, slowly clarifying and naming the affects, and including identification of the therapist's contribution to the break. The focus remains on the mind rather than on behavior, relating affects to the current event or activity and the "mental reality," using the therapist's mind as a model with the option of disclosure (option C). Transference-focused psychotherapy (option A) involves only individual sessions, does not focus on mentalization as exclusively as MBT, and involves early focus on the transference. Supportive-expressive therapy (option B) also does not involve group sessions, does not focus on mentalization as exclusively, and may involve early focus on the transference. Although certain approaches to psychoanalysis may focus on mentalization and may work toward achieving reflective functioning in the transference, psychoanalysis (option D) does not involve group sessions. **(pp. 230–232)**

10.6   According to the theory underlying MBT, which of the following early life conditions are related to later failures in mentalization?

A. Attunement difficulties between the infant and the caretaker impede a secure sense of attachment.
B. The child has a punitive superego.
C. The infant fails to integrate good and bad experiences of self and others.
D. Caregivers are not available to affirm, and to be idealized by, the child, who therefore does not develop a cohesive sense of self.
E. The child has a weak ego and uses primitive defenses.

The correct response is option A: Attunement difficulties between the infant and the caretaker impede a secure sense of attachment.

The theory underlying MBT attributes failures in mentalization to insecure attachment, resulting from deficiencies in infant-parent attunement during the patient's infancy. MBT restricts its emphasis to helping the patient repair failures in mentalizing without addressing the resolution of intrapsychic conflicts (options B, C, E). The therapist's efforts to increase the patient's capacity to mentalize help the patient move from a disorganized attachment, in which affects are volatile and unpredictable and the patient's subjectivity is vulnerable to collapse, toward a more secure attachment in which they are less capricious and more stable. Identifying and fostering appropriate expressions of affect is integral to this process. Within the range of affects, anger and aggression are seen as responses to neglect and abuse rather than primary affects that eventually need to be integrated into the self as a part of treatment (option D). **(p. 231)**

10.7   Which of the following best describes the relative roles of supportive techniques and expressive techniques in the major psychodynamic approaches to treating PDs?

A. All approaches to the psychodynamic treatment of PDs prioritize expressive techniques over supportive techniques.

B. Some approaches to the psychodynamic treatment of PDs emphasize expressive techniques over supportive techniques, some emphasize supportive techniques over expressive techniques, and some emphasize a mix of supportive and expressive techniques.
C. All approaches to the psychodynamic treatment of PDs prioritize supportive techniques over expressive techniques.
D. All approaches to the psychodynamic treatment of PDs emphasize a mix of supportive and expressive techniques.
E. The distinction between supportive techniques and expressive techniques is less relevant to the psychodynamic treatment of patients with PDs than it is to the psychodynamic treatment of patients without PDs.

The correct response is option B: Some approaches to the psychodynamic treatment of PDs emphasize expressive techniques over supportive techniques, some emphasize supportive techniques over expressive techniques, and some emphasize a mix of supportive and expressive techniques.

Psychotherapy techniques derived from psychoanalysis, including clarification, confrontation, and interpretation, are called "expressive." Other techniques, including advice and praise, are described as "supportive." Psychoanalysis and TFP are examples of approaches that emphasize expressive techniques over supportive techniques. Psychodynamically informed supportive psychotherapy emphasizes mostly supportive interventions. In supportive-expressive therapy, the therapist chooses between supportive and expressive techniques based on assessment of the patient's needs at that moment. **(pp. 234–235)**

10.8   Which of the following modalities of psychodynamic psychotherapy for PDs involves twice-weekly meetings; a focus on the treatment contract prior to beginning treatment; and an emphasis on clarification, confrontation, and early interpretation of representations of self and others as they emerge in the transference?

A. MBT.
B. Supportive-expressive therapy.
C. TFP.
D. Psychoanalysis.
E. Supportive psychotherapy.

The correct response is option C: TFP.

TFP combines an emphasis on the structure of the treatment, established through the contracting process, which is not a feature of psychoanalysis (option D) or supportive-expressive therapy (option B). TFP uses the exploration of the patient's internal world of representations of self and others, which is not a feature of supportive psychotherapy (option E). TFP is a twice-weekly individual therapy emphasizing the therapist's empathy with the entire range of the patient's affective responses, including negative affects as they arise in the transference.

Addressing the negative transference early on is felt to create a fuller alliance with the patient by indicating that the therapist can tolerate, and help the patient tolerate, the expression of the patient's most difficult internal states in order to move on to helping integrate those states with the aid of the interpretive process. MBT does not take this approach to negative aspects of the doctor-patient relationship (option A). **(p. 229)**

10.9   Which of the following is true of the evidence basis for psychodynamic treatment of PDs?

A. Across diagnoses, evidence supporting the use of cognitive-behavioral therapy (CBT) far outweighs evidence supporting the use of psychodynamic psychotherapy.
B. There is little empirical evidence that psychodynamic psychotherapy is useful in the treatment of PDs.
C. Transference interpretations, which are central to psychoanalytic or psychodynamic psychotherapy, have been shown to be most effective with psychologically minded patients and least effective with patients who are not psychologically minded.
D. Several modalities of psychodynamic psychotherapy have been demonstrated to be effective in the treatment of PDs.
E. TFP has been found to be less effective than either DBT or supportive psychotherapy when treating patients with PDs who are not psychologically minded.

The correct response is option D: Several modalities of psychodynamic psychotherapy have been demonstrated to be effective in the treatment of PDs.

In the overall field of psychotherapy, since the 1990s there has been an increasing emphasis on evidence-based treatments. There exists a misunderstanding that the body of evidence for CBT treatments far outweighs that for psychodynamic treatments (option A). A series of meta-analyses (see Shedler 2010 for a review) has corrected that misunderstanding (option B). Psychotherapy research is a broad field. The most publicized studies to date involve randomized controlled trials designed to compare a model of treatment with a control to establish the efficacy of treatment. However, an emerging area of research investigates the impact of specific elements within a therapy. An example of this is Høglend et al.'s (2008) work that studied transference interpretations in contrast to interpretations that do not address the transference. His findings turned traditional clinical thinking on its head: transference interpretations were found to have the most impact on patients who were at a lower level of self-other relatedness (option C). TFP was found to be particularly good for patients with low mentalizing capacities compared with DBT or supportive psychotherapy (option E). **(pp. 219–220)**

10.10 The related concepts of object relations dyads and internal working models are derived from which of the theoretical schools listed below?

A. Object relations theory and attachment theory.
B. Self psychology and attachment theory.
C. Object relations theory and ego psychology.
D. Libido theory and ego psychology.
E. Attachment theory and ego psychology.

The correct response is option A: Object relations theory and attachment theory.

Central to attachment theory is the concept of internal working models or mental representations that are formed through repeated transactions with attachment figures (Bretherton 1987; Shaver et al. 1996). These working models subsequently act as heuristic guides in relationships, organizing personality development and the regulation of affect. They include expectations, beliefs, emotional appraisals, and rules for processing or excluding information. These working models are partly conscious and partly unconscious and need not be completely consistent or coherent. This is reminiscent of Kernberg's (1984) concept of the object relations dyad. The similarities speak to underlying conceptual similarities between object relations theory and attachment theory. For instance, although Bowlby (1973) stressed that internal working models "are tolerably accurate reflections of the experiences those individuals actually had" (p. 20), he also realized that internal working models could be distorted as Kernberg emphasized in arguing for the centrality of transference interpretation. Moreover, both object relations dyads and internal working models include representations of self and others that are complementary and mutually confirming and include unconscious and emotional aspects of representation. Both theories note that these representations need not be consistent or coherent and that, to the degree that multiple inconsistent representations exist, the individual will have difficulty behaving consistently. Both Kernberg and Bowlby note that these multiple and inconsistent representations could oscillate in the individual's consciousness. Both authors discuss defensive processes for excluding representational information that is difficult to integrate with conscious representations of self and others; Kernberg (1984) called this *splitting*, whereas Bowlby (1973) referred to this process as *defensive exclusion*. Object relations dyads and internal working models are less central to self psychology theory than is the cohesiveness and vitality versus weakness and fragmentation of the self (option B). Ego psychology focuses more centrally on defenses and on conflicts between id, ego, and superego than it does on the description of object relations dyads or internal working models (options C, E). Libido theory focuses more on drives than it does on object relations dyad or internal working models (option D). **(pp. 225–226)**

References

Bowlby J: Attachment and Loss, Vol. 2: Separation, Anxiety, and Anger. London, Hogarth Press and Institute of Psycho-Analysis, 1973

Bretherton I: New perspectives on attachment relations: security, communication, and internal working models, in Handbook of Infant Development, 2nd Edition. Edited by Osofsky JD. Oxford, UK, Wiley, 1987, pp 1061–1100

Høglend P, Bogwald KP, Amlo S, et al: Transference interpretations in dynamic psychotherapy: do they really yield sustained effects? Am J Psychiatry 165:763–771, 2008 18413707

Kernberg OF: Severe Personality Disorders: Psychotherapeutic Strategies. New Haven, CT, Yale University Press, 1984

Shaver PR, Collins N, Clark CL: Attachment styles and internal working models of self and relationship partners, in Knowledge Structures in Close Relationships: A Social Psychological Approach. Edited by Fletcher J. Hillsdale, NJ, Lawrence Erlbaum, 1996, pp 25–61

Shedler J: The efficacy of psychodynamic psychotherapy. Am Psychol 65:98–109, 2010 20141265

CHAPTER 11

Cognitive-Behavioral Therapy I: Basics and Principles

11.1 Which of the following represents a central therapeutic goal of contemporary cognitive-behavioral treatment for personality disorders (PDs)?

A. The therapist should seek to change the patient's basic assumptions and cognitions.
B. The therapist should assist the patient in linking mood fluctuations to interpersonal situations.
C. The therapist should encourage patients to practice goal-oriented behavior in the face of dysfunctional cognitions.
D. The therapist should guide the patient toward uncovering the role of unconscious conflict in maintaining maladaptive behaviors.
E. The therapist should guide the patient away from any psychopharmacologic treatments.

The correct response is option C: The therapist should encourage patients to practice goal-oriented behavior in the face of dysfunctional cognitions.

Traditional cognitive-behavioral approaches are based on the concept that dysfunctional and maladaptive thinking play a major role in the etiology and persistence of PDs. Two major dimensions have extended the traditional field of cognitive-behavioral therapy (CBT) in recent years and have influenced the conceptualization of psychosocial treatments focusing on PDs: 1) the increasing importance of emotions and emotion regulation as outlined in dialectical behavior therapy (DBT) (Linehan et al. 2007) and 2) the importance of metacognitive processing as manifested in the so-called third wave of CBT (e.g., acceptance and commitment therapy [Hayes and Smith 2005]) (Wells 2003). Thus modern CBT no longer primarily aims to change patients' maladaptive beliefs, automatic thoughts, and related behavior (option A). Currently, contemporary cognitive-behavioral therapists for PDs encourage patients to learn to observe their emotions and cognitions from a metacognitive perspective, accept them as they are, anticipate the impact of action tendencies on short- and long-term goals, and learn how to practice goal-oriented behavior in the face of dysfunctional cognitions. Although a focus on interpersonal contexts (option B) is an important element of CBT, it is not the main tenet of the treatment. This is a characteristic goal of interpersonal psychotherapy (IPT) for borderline PD (BPD). Elucidation of unconscious conflict (option D) is the core feature of psychoanalytic or psychodynamic therapy. Treatment with CBT does not preclude use of medications (option E). **(p. 241)**

11.2   Empirically validated treatment recommendations currently exist for which of the following PDs?

A. Narcissistic.
B. Obsessive-compulsive.
C. Histrionic.
D. Avoidant.
E. Schizoid.

The correct response is option D: Avoidant.

Empirically validated treatment recommendations currently exist for only three specific PDs: borderline, antisocial, and avoidant. Although therapists generally treat other PDs, empirically validated treatments for narcissistic PD, obsessive-compulsive PD, histrionic PD, and schizoid PD do not yet exist (options A, B, C, E). **(pp. 241, 246)**

11.3   Which of the following factors is *most* relevant to consider when planning cognitive-behavioral treatment for a patient with a PD?

A. External social variables.
B. Family history of suicide.
C. Prior medication trials.
D. Prior psychiatric admissions.
E. Insurance and financial resources.

The correct response is option A: External social variables.

Treatment planning for CBT of patients with PDs should at least consider the following relevant components: individual expectations, values, and aims of the patient; current psychosocial status of the patient; individual characteristics of the patient; disorder-specific prototypical behavioral and experiential patterns; co-occurring other psychiatric disorders; co-occurring physical disorders; and external social variables (see Table 11–1 provided below). Options B, C, D, and E are important factors to consider when embarking on any form of psychiatric treatment for patients with PDs but are not specifically pertinent to cognitive-behavioral treatment planning. **(pp. 246–247)**

Key elements of treatment planning for patients with personality disorders

- Socioeconomic status
- Treatment history
- Individual expectations, values, and aims of the patient
- Potential treatment confounders
  - Suicidality
  - Behavior control
  - Co-occurring psychiatric disorders
  - Co-occurring somatic disorders
  - External social problems
- Problem analysis

11.4   A 27-year-old woman with BPD is in weekly psychotherapy. Her therapist goes on vacation for 2 weeks, during which time the patient experiences a recurrence of self-injurious behavior. How would a cognitive-behavioral therapist describe this patient's behavior?

A. Goal-related behavior.
B. Transference reaction.
C. Treatment-interfering behavior.
D. Acting-out behavior.
E. Crisis-generating behavior.

The correct response is option E: Crisis-generating behavior.

When treating patients with PDs, cognitive-behavioral therapists consider the "dynamic treatment hierarchy" proposed by Linehan (1993). At the top of this hierarchy is severe *crisis-generating behavior* (acute suicidality, severe aggressive outbursts, life-threatening parasuicidal behavior, etc.). These types of behaviors are always to be treated as a primary focus if present. The second tier of the dynamic treatment hierarchy concerns patterns of behavior that endanger the therapeutic relationship or maintenance of the treatment (i.e., *treatment-interfering behavior,* option C). Examples of treatment-interfering behavior include frequent cancellations or missed appointments and repeatedly coming late to sessions. *Goal-related behavior* (option A) is the final target of the treatment hierarchy, which relates to attainment of the treatment goals. *Transference reaction* (option B) is a term utilized by psychodynamic psychotherapists to describe unconscious redirection of feelings toward the therapist. *Acting out* (option D) is another psychoanalytic term that refers to patients who engage in extreme behaviors to express conflicts and feelings that they are otherwise unable to recognize within themselves or to verbalize. **(p. 248)**

11.5   After several months of CBT, a 35-year-old man with avoidant PD decides to attend a social gathering. Fifteen minutes into the party he leaves because he thinks the other guests find him awkward and inadequate. How would a cognitive-behavioral therapist describe this phenomenon?

A. Defense against anticipated rejection.
B. Dysfunctional misinterpretation.
C. Anxiety over dependency needs.
D. Interpersonal deficits.
E. Avoidant attachment style.

The correct response is option B: Dysfunctional misinterpretation.

The cognitive-behavioral theory of PDs is based on the concept that such patients tend to process information according to filters that may be highly selective or biased. Patients with PDs tend to appraise situations in a way that is exaggerated or dysfunctional, although they do not usually perceive these assessments as problematic. Cognitive-behavioral therapists seek to help patients with PDs recognize these prototypic dysfunctional interpretation patterns, anticipate the impact of these tendencies on short- and long-term goals, and find a way to engage in meaningful goal-oriented behavior in the face of distorted emotions and cognitions. Options A and C are psychodynamic conceptualizations of avoidant personality, whereas option E is a formulation of avoidant behavior rooted in attachment theory rather than the cognitive-behavioral model. Interpersonal deficits (option D) refers to a common focus of IPT rather than a CBT model. **(pp. 241–242, 249–250)**

11.6   Which of the following is a true statement about psychoeducation in the cognitive-behavioral treatment of patients with PDs?

A. Patients should not be told their diagnosis because it will increase risk of suicide.
B. Patients have a right to be told their diagnosis, and concealing this information is an ethical violation.
C. Informing patients with PDs about their diagnosis is a straightforward aspect of psychoeducation that is rarely debated.
D. Only patients with Cluster C PDs should be informed of their diagnosis.
E. For selected PDs, the benefits of openly communicating the diagnosis mostly outweigh the disadvantages.

The correct response is option E: For selected PDs, the benefits of openly communicating the diagnosis mostly outweigh the disadvantages.

Whether a patient with a PD should be informed about his or her diagnosis is a complex issue that has been the subject of controversial debate for many years (option C). Arguments against openly communicating the diagnosis include issues such as stigmatization and negative effects on the therapeutic relationship. Some practitioners may feel that discussion of the diagnosis is an essential component of disorder-specific psychotherapy. In general, cognitive-behavioral therapists tend to include discussion of the diagnosis as a flexible part of the general psychoeducational approach, in which informed and clear language is used to help to delineate the treatment model, destigmatize and demystify the diagnosis, and enhance treatment motivation. Using a resource- and problem-oriented view of the personality, additional information about diagnosis should be guided not solely by DSM-5 criteria (option D) but also by the individual thinking and unique experiences and patterns of the patient. There is no evidence to suggest that disclosure of diagnosis increases risk of suicide in patients with PDs (option A). Option B is also incorrect because one could make the ethical argument of therapeutic privilege (e.g., it is ethical to conceal information from patients about their condition if it is likely to cause them undue harm or suffering). **(pp. 252–253)**

11.7   Which of the following is true of therapy contracts in cognitive-behavioral treatment of patients with PDs?

A. Therapy contracts should include discussion of expected duration and frequency of treatment.
B. Discussion of suicidal crises and behavior is not typically addressed in cognitive-behavioral treatment contracts.
C. Patients with PDs should not be told how to reach the therapist in case of emergency because they are likely to abuse this privilege.
D. Therapy contracts for patients with PDs are no different than those for patients with other psychiatric diagnoses.
E. Patients with PDs should not be informed of the therapist's training and supervision.

The correct response is option A: Therapy contracts should include discussion of expected duration and frequency of treatment.

Clarification of the treatment frame, or of the general conditions of treatment, including discussion of expected duration and frequency of treatment, is a basic prerequisite for all psychotherapeutic interventions. In the treatment of patients with PDs, a number of special features need to be taken into consideration and appropriately addressed (option D). For example, suicidal crises are an expected part of treatment with such patients and should be explicitly addressed in the treatment contract (option B). Patients with PDs should also be given clear information about expected financial arrangements in addition to duration/frequency. It is often useful to tell the patient where and under which conditions the therapist can be reached in case of emergency (option C). Option E is incorrect because the patient does have a right to know how and by whom the therapist receives supervision and which materials are used in that process. **(p. 253)**

11.8   A 52-year-old man with narcissistic PD has been in regular CBT for 1 month and has developed a good therapeutic alliance. When his therapist is 10 minutes late for a session, the patient angrily says, "What a fool I am for thinking you were better than the rest of the world out there…turns out you are no different. …You are incompetent and of no use to me." Which of the following is the correct response for the therapist to make to the patient?

A. The therapist stays silent and expressionless, waiting to see what the patient will say next.
B. "You are being extremely rude. This behavior is unacceptable and I will be unable to continue the session if you cannot calm down."
C. "I am sorry that I was late. I see that you are angry and with good reason. Nevertheless, your behavior right now is making me feel rather helpless. Is that your intention?"
D. "I am sorry that I was late. Tell me what it felt like to be kept waiting."
E. "You are clearly feeling hurt and disappointed, and I think you are taking that out on me to punish me and make me feel what you are feeling. This is what you do with the rest of the world, and it is why you are so alone and miserable."

The correct response is option C: "I am sorry that I was late. I see that you are angry and with good reason. Nevertheless, your behavior right now is making me feel rather helpless. Is that your intention?"

Cognitive-behavioral therapists often observe dysfunctional verbal or behavioral patterns in sessions with patients who have PDs. These situations can provide an invaluable substrate in which the therapeutic relationship can be examined and employed as a source of change. Some common cognitive-behavioral techniques that therapists use for this purpose include describing and validating the observed behavior as well as telling the patient their own cognitive or emotional reaction to the behavior. See Table 11–3 provided below. Option A is an example of absolute therapeutic neutrality, which is more likely to be used in a psychoanalytic treatment in order to foster free association or transference neurosis. Option B is a judgmental statement and unlikely to be of therapeutic utility. Option D is a supportive intervention in which the therapist aims to get at the patient's inner psychic experience of rejection and disappointment. This kind of inquiry is more typically used in psychodynamic treatments as opposed to CBT. Although option E may be a correct explanation of what is going on in the therapeutic relationship, it is a premature statement that does not allow the patient to recognize what he or she is feeling or generate alternative behavioral strategies for coping with his emotions. **(pp. 255–256)**

A clinical algorithm to use for in-session observations for behavioral change

1. Observe dysfunctional verbal or behavioral in-session patterns and observe your emotional reactions (e.g., patient looks hostile and falls into silence after reporting suicidal thoughts).
2. Ask the patient whether feedback is desired: "May I give you some short feedback?"
3. Describe the behavior observed and validate:
"It seems to me that you have become silent and look quite angry after telling me your suicidal thoughts. If I am right, I am sure that you have good reasons for how you're feeling. Is that right?"
4. Describe your own cognitive or emotional reaction:
"Nevertheless, your behavior makes me feel quite helpless and anxious."

A clinical algorithm to use for in-session observations for behavioral change *(continued)*

5. Ask whether your reaction is intended by the patient:
   "Is this your intention?"

6. If the patient denies it (as is typical), then ask for the "real" intention:
   "Fine, so what is your intention?"

7. Whatever the patient answers, help the patient process intentions adequately:
   "Oh, you feel helpless by yourself and you expect clear advice from me, such as how to cope with suicidal thoughts? That makes sense to me—so please try to think about and tell me what your expectations are, because otherwise we might run into trouble."

8. Link functional behavior to the individual goals of the patient:
   "…and by the way…it might be not entirely useless to learn how to ask for concrete help and advice—perhaps regarding your wish to continue your fellowship program in May."

9. Do not forget to shape functional behavior:
   "This time it seems to me that you directly ask for advice about the skills needed to take that step, and it looks like an effort to change your communication style—which is one of the goals we've been working on. Is that correct?"

11.9   Which of the following is an exercise that a patient in CBT may practice in order to help identify dysfunctional information processing?

   A. Mindfulness meditation.
   B. Analysis of transference.
   C. Interpersonal inventory.
   D. Behavioral or chain analysis.
   E. Dream analysis.

The correct response is option D: Behavioral or chain analysis.

Behavioral or *chain analysis* is a functional form of behavioral analysis rooted in behavioral psychology that can help patients observe maladaptive cognitive responses. It is used in cognitive and dialectical behavioral therapy for patients with PDs. Option B (analysis of transference) and option E (dream analysis) are psychoanalytic techniques. Interpersonal inventory (option C) is a key method used in IPT to help patients take stock of interpersonal dysfunction and understand their illness within an interpersonal context. Although CBT certainly seeks to help patients increase mindfulness (option A), meditation is not usually a standard part of this treatment for PDs. **(pp. 256–257)**

11.10   A 47-year-old woman with paranoid PD is in weekly CBT. She tells her therapist that her coworker has been more aloof lately and is "probably getting cozy with the boss to try to edge me out and make me look bad." Which of the following would be a correct CBT response?

   A. "You sound very angry at your coworker; I think you are projecting your hostility."
   B. "Could there be another possible explanation for your coworker's recent behavior?"

C. "You are using the cognitive distortion of 'mind reading.' Let's try to change that."

D. "It sounds like you feel threatened by your coworker. What comes to mind about that?"

E. "You are responding to your coworker the same way you did to your sister growing up when you felt excluded and inferior."

The correct response is option B: "Could there be another possible explanation for your coworker's recent behavior?"

Cognitive-behavioral therapists seek to help their patients identify dysfunctional information processing and clarify the consequences of these thoughts on an emotional and behavioral level. *Cognitive restructuring* is a core technique used to help emphasize problematic automatic thoughts and carefully help the patient explore alternative perspectives. Option C correctly identifies one of the patient's dysfunctional cognitions about her coworker. However, the therapist preemptively attempts to change the patient's basic assumption before allowing the patient to learn to recognize her own emotions and cognitions first. Option A is a premature interpretation of a defense. Interpretation of defenses is a technique that would most likely be used in psychodynamic psychotherapy. Option D is an open-ended response intended to foster free association on the part of the patient and would also be found in psychoanalytic or psychodynamic treatments. Option E is a genetic interpretation about early life relationship templates that may be influencing the patient's current emotional reaction and view of herself and others. Although cognitive-behavioral therapists are certainly interested in such long-standing core beliefs or assumptions (referred to as "schemas"), direct interpretation making links to the distant past is not a common feature of CBT. Rather, this is more likely to be utilized by a psychoanalytically or psychodynamically oriented therapist. **(pp. 256–257)**

References

Hayes S, Smith S: Get Out of Your Mind and Into Your Life: The New Acceptance and Commitment Therapy. Oakland, CA, New Harbinger Publications, 2005

Linehan M: Cognitive-Behavioral Treatment of Borderline Personality Disorder. New York, Guilford, 1993

Linehan MM, Bohus M, Lynch T: Dialectical behavior therapy for pervasive emotion dysregulation: theoretical and practical underpinnings, in Handbook of Emotion Regulation. Edited by Gross J. New York, Guilford, 2007, pp 581–605

Wells A: Emotional Disorders and Metacognition: Innovative Cognitive Therapy. Hoboken, NJ, Wiley, 2003

CHAPTER 1 2

Cognitive-Behavioral Therapy II: Specific Strategies for Personality Disorders

12.1 What does the cognitive-behavioral therapy (CBT) technique of cognitive restructuring emphasize in the treatment of patients with personality disorders (PDs)?

A. How the thought process functions within the person's life.
B. The content of the negative thoughts.
C. Preventing nonsuicidal self-injury (NSSI).
D. Relationship to managing negative emotions.
E. Irrational thoughts without consideration to context.

The correct response is option A: How the thought process functions within the person's life.

With PDs, the context by which the negative thoughts and beliefs affect interpersonal, emotional, and cognitive domains is critical to treatment. In addition, contextual factors related to maladaptive thoughts are thought to reinforce both maladaptive behavior and negative emotions. Furthermore, maintaining therapeutic alliance is especially critical for CBT with PDs. Many patients experience or have experienced their environment as invalidating. Therefore, it is important for therapists to be empathic and understanding of how thought processes developed versus conceptualizing thoughts as irrational (option E). Also, challenging the maladaptive thought extends beyond examining the content of a belief (option B). In addition, targeting self-destructive and defeating behaviors (option C) and affect dysregulation (option D) is assumed to be necessary to work with patients with PDs; however, neither are critical to CBT interventions. **(pp. 261–262)**

12.2 In using CBT with patients with PDs, what is the most important feature of setting treatment goals?

A. Flexibility.
B. Collaboration.
C. Noncritical statements.
D. Focusing on interpersonal relationships.
E. Addressing nonsuicidal self-injurious behavior.

The correct response is option B: Collaboration.

Establishing individualized treatment goals while creating a solid therapeutic alliance is critical to CBT in general. When treating PDs, treatment goals should be a collaborative negotiation to best maintain the therapeutic alliance, which is imperative. Agreement is likely to increase motivation. Flexibility (option A) is important in this ongoing, fluid process, in which collaboratively planned interventions are intended to become part of patient's way of experiencing the world, but it is not critical to setting treatment goals. Noncritical statements (option C), focusing on interpersonal relationships (option D), and addressing nonsuicidal behavior (option E) are helpful when providing CBT to patients with PDs, but they are also not critical to setting treatment goals. **(pp. 261–262)**

12.3 A 25-year-old female patient presents with symptoms consistent with borderline PD (BPD). She reports that her greatest concern, and reason for seeking treatment, is unstable relationships with men, friends, and family. Her father has always been verbally abusive and her mother has been emotionally unavailable because of severe depression. The patient experiences her early and current home environment as critical and invalidating. She has developed a view of herself as worthless and a view of others as rejecting. When she perceives rejection, she is prone to intense anger, acting impulsively or engaging in nonsuicidal self-injurious behavior. On the basis of the research and her beliefs about self and others, which type of CBT should be considered and will likely be most effective?

A. Acceptance and commitment therapy.
B. Dialectical behavior therapy (DBT).
C. Schema-focused therapy (SFT).
D. Mindfulness-based treatment.
E. Cognitive-analytic therapy.

The correct response is option C: Schema-focused therapy (SFT).

The patient's early maladaptive beliefs related to self and others are called *schemas*, which trigger and maintain interpersonal difficulties. This is the primary focus of SFT. In addition, a large-scale randomized controlled trial has shown that SFT lessens relationship impairment, identity problems, impulsivity, and NSSI (Giesen-Bloo et al. 2006), all of which are endorsed by this patient. DBT (option B) has been shown to effectively treat BPD; however, this type of CBT focuses more on current functioning by targeting maladaptive behaviors (e.g., NSSI) and emotion regulation. SFT as compared with DBT involves working through underlying psychological constructs that trigger painful experiences and that formed early in development. Acceptance and commitment therapy, mindfulness-based treatment, and cognitive-analytic therapy (options A, D, E) are new therapeutic approaches and require further research to determine effectiveness for PDs. **(pp. 262, 265–266)**

12.4   For which PD has research shown modest effects for CBT but not demonstrated superiority over treatment as usual (TAU)?

    A. Dependent PD.
    B. Schizotypal PD.
    C. BPD.
    D. Histrionic PD.
    E. Antisocial PD.

The correct response is option E: Antisocial PD.

CBT for antisocial PD has demonstrated decreases in aggressive behavior but no improvements in depression, anxiety, anger, or negative beliefs about others. In general, no psychological interventions for antisocial PD have emerged as effective, which is thought to be due to poor prognostic indicators such as attachment difficulties (i.e., inability to form working therapeutic alliance), narcissism, and limited emotional development. Several studies exist to establish that CBT for BPD has been shown to be more effective than TAU (option C). To date, no known open trials or randomized control trials exist that assess CBT for treatment of dependent (option A), schizotypal (option B), or histrionic (option D) PDs. **(p. 265)**

12.5   What is a newer form of CBT that is currently being explored and adapted to treatment of PDs?

    A. DBT.
    B. Psychodynamic therapy.
    C. Acceptance and commitment therapy.
    D. Interpersonal therapy.
    E. SFT.

The correct response is option C: Acceptance and commitment therapy.

Acceptance and commitment therapy is part of a new wave of cognitive-behavioral interventions that use acceptance and mindfulness strategies to decrease psychological symptoms. Given the empirical evidence on the effectiveness for several disorders, the application of this approach to PDs is being developed and tested. DBT (option A), interpersonal psychotherapy (option D), and SFT (option E) are well-established forms of CBT. Psychodynamic therapy (option B) is also a well-established intervention that is separate and distinct from CBT. **(p. 268)**

12.6 Therapist effects were found to be significant in the Borderline Personality Disorder Study of Cognitive Therapy, a well-designed randomized clinical trial to test efficacy of CBT (Davidson et al. 2006). With which of the following provided by the therapists did patients have two to three times greater improvement in suicide-related outcomes?

A. Emergency services and medication management.
B. Cognitive techniques to modify core beliefs and schemas.
C. Behavioral strategies to promote adaptive functioning.
D. Higher quantity and more competent delivery of CBT.
E. Exposure to situations that triggered emotional distress.

The correct response is option D: Higher quantity and more competent delivery of CBT.

Because the active treatment group did not show improvements in psychiatric hospitalizations or emergency department admissions compared with the TAU group, therapist effects were analyzed and found to impact treatment efficacy. Specifically, both higher quantity of sessions and more competent delivery as assessed by a competence rating scale related to greater improvement in suicide-related outcomes (Norrie et al. 2013). In the active treatment group, all therapists provided cognitive techniques to modify core beliefs and schemas (option B) and behavioral strategies to promote adaptive functioning (option C). Therapists may have provided exposure to situations that triggered emotional distress (option E), which is a component of CBT treatment, but this specific technique was not a standard part of this protocol. In the TAU group, only emergency services and medication management were provided (option A). **(p. 263)**

12.7 What is a major difference between DBT and traditional CBT?

A. Maladaptive behaviors are viewed with acceptance and validation.
B. Historical context is considered in the development of negative cognitions.
C. Solid empirical evidence exists to support effectiveness.
D. NSSI is monitored and addressed.
E. Skills training is emphasized.

The correct response is option A: Maladaptive behaviors are viewed with acceptance and validation.

Although DBT is considered a type of CBT, an important distinction exists with respect to maladaptive behavior. DBT is based on Linehan's (1993) biopsychosocial theory of BPD. The theory proposes that emotional and behavioral dysregulation are elicited and reinforced by the interplay between an invalidating developmental environment and individual biological tendencies toward emotional reactivity. Therefore, maladaptive behaviors are understandable reactions to environmental triggers and are approached with acceptance and validation. In traditional CBT, maladaptive behaviors are considered dysfunctional and unproductive as well as a result of inaccurate cognitions and negative emotions. Both DBT and CBT are similar in that the historical context is considered in the development of negative cognitions (option B), empirical evidence exists to support effectiveness (option C), and skills training is emphasized (option E). With DBT only, NSSI is monitored and addressed (option D), but this feature is not considered a major difference between traditional CBT. **(p. 266)**

12.8 What did the results of randomized clinical trials consistently show for group-based cognitive-behavioral treatments for PDs?

A. Significant reduction of NSSI behavior.
B. Superiority over TAU.
C. No difference as compared with TAU.
D. Greater effectiveness as compared with psychodynamic therapy.
E. Equally as effective as individual CBT.

The correct response is option B: Superiority over TAU.

Group-based cognitive-behavioral treatments for PDs were shown to be superior to TAU. This finding was consistent across all four randomized clinical trials (Blum et al. 2008; Freije et al. 2002; Gratz and Gunderson 2006; Van Wel et al. 2006). Specifically, the treatment groups that received Systems Training for Emotional Predictability and Problem Solving or Emotion Regulation Group Therapy showed decreased BPD symptomatology (e.g., emotional dysregulation, negative emotions such as depression and anxiety) compared with the TAU group. **(pp. 264–265)**

12.9 Which of the models used in DSM-5 for PDs best matches with a CBT treatment approach?

A. Dimensional model.
B. Categorical model.
C. Cluster trait model.
D. Quantitative hierarchical model.
E. Hybrid Axis I and II model.

The correct response is option A: Dimensional model.

The dimensional model of PDs is consistent with a CBT approach in that both focus on problematic areas of functioning. According to research and to Section III, "Emerging Measures and Models," of DSM-5, PDs are best organized using a dimensional model, in which a single diagnostic concept is used to communicate a large amount of integrated clinical information. Cognitive-behavioral treatments have been developed to treat specific diagnostic concepts (e.g., anxiety, depression, insomnia, trauma) that overlap with multiple disorders and, therefore, match the dimensional model. The inclusion of the dimensional model in DSM-5 Section III came about because of the major limitations of a categorical model (option B) such as excessive co-occurrence among disorders, extreme heterogeneity among patients receiving the same diagnosis, and arbitrary diagnostic thresholds for distinguishing pathological and "normal" personality functioning. The dimensional model of personality psychopathology is designed to increase clinical utility and improve patient care. The cluster trait model (option C) is the organizing approach for the DSM-IV, not for the DSM-5. The quantitative hierarchical model (option D) uses empirical evidence to categorize disorders and is not the organizing approach for PDs in DSM-5. The Hybrid Axis I and II model (option E) is the organizing approach for all disorders in DSM-5 and is not specific to PDs. **(p. 262)**

12.10 Which of the following describes the current American Psychiatric Association (APA) treatment guideline for patients with BPD?

A. Pharmacotherapy only.
B. Primary treatment of pharmacotherapy with adjunctive psychotherapy.
C. Primary treatment of CBT.
D. Primary treatment of psychotherapy with adjunctive, symptom-targeted pharmacotherapy.
E. Pharmacotherapy with psychotherapy for anxiety, depressive, or substance abuse disorders as indicated.

The correct response is option D: Primary treatment of psychotherapy with adjunctive, symptom-targeted pharmacotherapy.

According to the American Psychiatric Association (2001) guideline for the treatment of patients with BPD, psychotherapy is needed to attain and maintain lasting improvement in their personality, interpersonal problems, and overall functioning. Therefore, psychotherapy is considered the primary treatment (option B). Pharmacotherapy alone (option A) is not considered the most effective treatment but a recent meta-analysis has shown it plays an important adjunctive role in decreasing the severity of anger, anxiety, impulsivity, psychotic-like symptoms, and self-destructive behavior (Ingenhoven et al. 2010). Therefore, the APA consensus is that patients will benefit most from a combination of these treatments. Primary treatment of CBT specifically (option C) is not recommended because a persuasive review of data from approximately 24 randomized controlled trials of BPD demonstrated clear and compelling evidence that several forms of psychotherapy, including CBT and dialectical behavior therapy, help patients with BPD. Pharmacotherapy with psychotherapy for anxiety, depressive, or substance abuse disorders (option E) does not address the defining features of PD (overarching pattern of distorted and maladaptive thinking about oneself and impaired interpersonal relationships). **(pp. 262–263)**

References

American Psychiatric Association: Practice guideline for the treatment of patients with borderline personality disorder. Am J Psychiatry 158 (10 suppl):1–52, 2001 11665545

Blum N, St. John D, Pfohl B, et al: Systems Training for Emotional Predictability and Problem Solving (STEPPS) for outpatients with borderline personality disorder: a randomized controlled trial and 1-year follow-up. Am J Psychiatry 165:468–478, 2008 18281407

Davidson K, Norrie J, Tyrer P, et al: The effectiveness of cognitive behavior therapy for borderline personality disorder: results from the borderline personality disorder study of cognitive therapy (BOSCOT) trial. J Pers Disord 20:450–465, 2006 17032158

Freije H, Dietz B, Appelo M: Borderline persoonlijkheidsstoornis met de VERS: de vaardigheidstraining emotionele regulatiestoornis. Directieve Therapie 4:367–378, 2002

Giesen-Bloo J, van Dyck R, Spinhoven P, et al: Outpatient psychotherapy for borderline personality disorder: randomized trial of schema-focused therapy vs transference-focused psychotherapy. Arch Gen Psychiatry 63:649–658, 2006 16754838

Gratz K, Gunderson J: Preliminary data on acceptance-based emotion regulation group intervention for deliberate self-harm among women with borderline personality disorder. Behav Ther 37:25–35, 2006 16942958

Linehan M: Cognitive-Behavioral Treatment of Borderline Personality Disorder. New York, Guilford, 1993

Norrie J, Davidson K, Tata P, et al: Influence of therapist competence and quantity of cognitive behavioural therapy on suicidal behaviour and inpatient hospitalisation in a randomised controlled trial in borderline personality disorder: further analyses of treatment effects in the BOSCOT study. Psychol Psychother 86:280–293, 2013 23420622

Van Wel B, Kockmann I, Blum N, et al: STEPPS group treatment for borderline personality disorder in the Netherlands. Ann Clin Psychiatry 18:63–67, 2006 16517455

CHAPTER 13

Group, Family, and Couples Therapies

13.1 What feature of personality disorders (PDs) makes group therapy, with its frequent verbal and nonverbal exchanges with others, particularly effective?

A. Patients are frequently oblivious to their interpersonal maladaptive behaviors.
B. Patients may have intrapersonal difficulties.
C. Patients may be prone to emotional outbursts.
D. Patients with self-injurious behaviors can benefit from expressing threats of harmful behavior.
E. Aggressive or threatening behaviors are mitigated in the group setting.

The correct response is option A: Patients are frequently oblivious to their interpersonal maladaptive behaviors.

Group therapy is especially effective in treating PDs when the patient is oblivious to his or her maladaptive behavior. The nature of group therapy allows for interpersonal maladaptive personality traits to be uncovered through intensive verbal and nonverbal interchanges within the group. Thus intrapersonal features of a PD are not particularly targeted within a group setting (option B). Patients who have emotional outbursts, make suicidal threats, or are aggressive toward other group members may not be appropriate for group therapy (options C, D, E). **(p. 282)**

13.2 How do patients with PDs more typically reveal their pathology, which may facilitate group treatment?

A. Describing in words.
B. Demonstrating in action.
C. Dealing with internally.
D. Defending against subconsciously.
E. Deliberating carefully.

The correct response is option B: Demonstrating in action.

Patients with PDs are more likely than patients with various other psychiatric illness to demonstrate their pathology in interpersonal exchanges than to describe it in words or keep the pathology to themselves, making group therapy especially useful. **(p. 283)**

13.3   Which PDs are associated with the role of therapist helper in the group therapy setting?

A. Antisocial PD and narcissistic PD.
B. Dependent PD and histrionic PD.
C. Paranoid PD and avoidant PD.
D. Obsessive-compulsive PD and borderline PD (BPD).
E. Schizoid PD and schizotypal PD.

The correct response is option B: Dependent PD and histrionic PD.

Patients with dependent and histrionic PDs often assume a therapist helper role in the group setting. **(p. 283)**

13.4   What is the role of the therapist when a patient is identified as a difficult group member?

A. Ask the patient to leave the group.
B. Discern whether the individual may be serving a defensive function for the group.
C. Ask the patient during the group why he or she is being difficult so that the group can contribute to the discussion.
D. Avoid bringing attention to the problem so that the patient's feelings are not hurt.
E. Invite the patient to join an alternative group to see if the problems continue.

The correct response is option B: Discern whether the individual may be serving a defensive function for the group.

At times "difficult" patients can engage in behaviors that serve a defensive function for the group, and a role of the therapist is to determine whether this is occurring. Asking a patient to leave the group (option A) may not resolve the problem if the individual is serving a defensive function for the group. Care should be taken not to further "scapegoat" an individual during the group by identifying him or her as "difficult" (option C); however, difficult behavior should not be ignored if it is impairing the group's ability to function (option D). Asking the patient to join another group (option E) will not ameliorate the problem if the individual's behavior is serving a defensive function for the group. **(pp. 283–284)**

13.5   What PD was the Systems Training for Emotional Predictability and Problem Solving (STEPPS) group therapy initially designed to target?

A. Narcissistic PD.
B. Histrionic PD.
C. Dependent PD.
D. Avoidant PD.
E. BPD.

The correct response is option E: BPD.

STEPPS (Blum et al. 2008) was originally designed as an adjunctive treatment program for patients with BPD. This therapy may be useful for other PDs but was originally designed for and studied in the borderline population. STEPPS group therapy includes a 2-hour weekly group seminar organized around specific emotional, cognitive, and behavioral self-management skills, as well as a psychoeducation group for key members of the patients' support networks. **(p. 284)**

13.6   What is the definition in terms of duration for long-term outpatient group therapy?

A. 12 weeks.
B. 6 months.
C. 1 year.
D. 2 years.
E. 3 years.

The correct response is option C: 1 year.

Long-term group therapy is usually defined as lasting a minimum of 1 year but may last longer. It is intensive in nature and, over time, involves confrontation and interpretation of the patient's core conflicts, defensive style, and long-term maladaptive behaviors. It attempts to modify the core traits and personality structure that characterize PDs. **(p. 284)**

13.7   In what way has dialectical behavioral therapy (DBT) been shown to be superior with respect to the following to treatment as usual?

A. Suicidal and self-injurious behaviors.
B. Distress.
C. Interpersonal problems.
D. Regulation of emotion.
E. Mindfulness.

The correct response is option A: Suicidal and self-injurious behaviors.

DBT has been shown to reduce suicidal and self-injurious behavior with patients with BPD. This therapy targets these behaviors by teaching a series of skills including distress tolerance, interpersonal effectiveness, emotion regulation, and mindfulness. **(p. 286)**

13.8   Which psychoanalytically oriented day treatment program combines group and individual therapy and is unique in the long follow-up period studied?

A. DBT.
B. Mentalization-based therapy.
C. Cognitive-behavioral therapy (CBT).
D. STEPPS.
E. Interpersonal psychotherapy.

The correct response is option B: Mentalization-based therapy.

Bateman and Fonagy (1999) developed mentalization-based therapy as a psychoanalytically oriented day treatment program that consists of a combination of group and individual therapies for 5 days per week for a maximum of 18 months. DBT (option A) typically includes individual psychotherapy, a skills group, and the opportunity for therapist coaching between sessions. CBT (option C) may be delivered in individual or group settings but is not by design a day treatment program. STEPPS (option D) is a group-based therapy. Interpersonal psychotherapy (option E) is an individual therapy. While DBT, CBT, STEPPS, and interpersonal psychotherapy are all evidence-based psychotherapies, mentalization-based therapy is unique in that it has been studied with a longer follow-up period than other psychotherapies. **(pp. 286–287)**

13.9   In which of the following situations might family therapy for treatment of a PD be contraindicated?

A. Family consists of more than five individuals.
B. Family includes more than one member with a PD.
C. Family includes a member who feels overwhelming embarrassment when discussing personal issues in front of family.
D. Family includes a member who is in individual therapy.
E. Family has multiple interpersonal difficulties.

The correct response is option C: Family includes a member who feels overwhelming embarrassment when discussing personal issues in front of family.

The therapist may need to assess whether family therapy may be contraindicated when one member of the family is not able to discuss problems without overwhelming embarrassment. Family therapy can be conducted with families of any size (option A) and can be especially helpful when multiple family members have mental illness (option B), when members are in individual therapy (option D), and when interpersonal difficulties exist (option E). **(p. 289)**

13.10 What is the effect of a positive romantic relationship on BPD?

A. No effect.
B. Healing effect.
C. Increased impulsivity.
D. Decreased functioning.
E. Increased regression.

The correct response is option B: Healing effect.

Research has demonstrated that a good marriage can have a healing effect on BPD characteristics in adulthood (Lewis 1998). Furthermore, marriage predicted better clinical outcome, improved functional status, and dampened levels of impulsivity (Links and Heslegrave 2000). **(p. 294)**

13.11 In DBT adapted for couples, dialectics include which of the following?

A. Intimacy versus autonomy.
B. Autonomy versus shame and doubt.
C. Intimacy versus isolation.
D. Trust versus mistrust.
E. Initiative versus guilt.

The correct response is option A: Intimacy versus autonomy.

Dialectics for couples therapy include 1) closeness versus conflict, 2) partner acceptance versus change, 3) one partner's needs versus the other's, 4) individual versus relationship satisfaction, and 5) intimacy versus autonomy. Autonomy versus shame and doubt, intimacy versus isolation, trust versus mistrust, and initiative versus guilt (options B, C, D, and E) are all psychosocial stages of development described by Erikson (1950). **(p. 297)**

References

Bateman A, Fonagy P: Effectiveness of partial hospitalization in the treatment of borderline personality disorder: a randomized controlled trial. Am J Psychiatry 156:1563–1569, 1999 10518167

Blum N, St. John D, Pfohl B, et al: Systems Training for Emotional Predictability and Problem Solving (STEPPS) for outpatients with borderline personality disorder: a randomized controlled trial and 1-year follow-up. Am J Psychiatry 165:468–478, 2008 18281407

Erikson EH: Childhood and Society. New York, WW Norton, 1950

Lewis JM: For better or worse: interpersonal relationships and individual outcome. Am J Psychiatry 155:582–589, 1998 9585706

Links PS, Heslegrave RJ: Prospective studies of outcome: understanding mechanisms of change in patients with borderline personality disorder. Psychiatr Clin North Am 23:137–150, 2000 10729936

CHAPTER 14

Psychoeducation

14.1 Which of the following statements comparing psychoeducation and psychotherapy is true?

A. As with psychotherapy, the methods and procedures of psychoeducation are both educational and therapeutic.
B. Psychotherapy has been shown to reduce recurrence, which is not true for psychoeducation.
C. Unlike psychotherapy, individuals in recovery or family members frequently deliver psychoeducation.
D. In contrast with psychotherapy, psychoeducation has yet to establish efficacy beyond Axis I disorders.
E. Psychoeducation, unlike psychotherapy, is evidence-based.

The correct response is option C: Unlike psychotherapy, individuals in recovery or family members frequently deliver psychoeducation.

Psychoeducation and psychotherapy are well-established, evidence-based practices for many psychiatric disorders. Numerous randomized clinical trials have demonstrated that psychoeducation programs help significantly reduce relapse and improve individual outcomes and the course of illness (options B, E). Both psychoeducation and psychotherapy have established efficacy in Axis I and Axis II disorders (option D). Psychoeducation is distinct from psychotherapy because the methods and procedures are entirely educational (option A). Unlike psychotherapy, psychoeducation is frequently delivered by individuals in recovery, family members, or by professionals without psychotherapy training. **(p. 303)**

14.2 Which focus of psychoeducation is thought to be most relevant to short-term and long-term patient outcomes?

A. Current family functioning factors.
B. Knowledge base alone.
C. Specific etiologic pathways for personality disorder (PD).
D. Existing treatment options, including medications and therapy.
E. Developmental history of the patient.

The correct response is option A: Current family functioning factors.

The best data available suggest that current family functioning factors are very relevant to both short- and long-term patient outcomes and thus should be a focus of psychoeducation. The data suggest that knowledge alone does not improve outcomes (option B); education may require the additional and complementary component of skill acquisition to have a significant impact. Despite wide acceptance of various theories, we do not know enough about the specific etiologic pathways for PD to make it a focus of psychoeducation (option C). Thoughtful professionals may reasonably interpret myriad studies in a variety of ways. What is clear is the heterogeneity of factors, including family interaction and family functioning, which may be found in the developmental histories of our patients. Thus being physically or sexually abused may be a risk factor for several PDs, yet the vast majority of survivors of physical and sexual abuse do not develop PDs. Similarly, having loving and attentive parents who do not have substance abuse or other mental health problems is a protective factor for most people. Yet some people with severe PDs have parents who fit this description. The current focus in the child development literature on transactional models (ongoing, reciprocal influence between individual psychological and biological factors and responses from parents and other caregivers) promises improved clarity about etiology in the future (options D, E) (Cummings et al. 2000; Eisenberg et al. 2003; Fruzzetti et al. 2005). **(pp. 306–307)**

14.3   Which core component is least consistently found in psychoeducational programs?

A. Education.
B. Problem solving.
C. Social support.
D. Skills training.
E. Bibliotherapy.

The correct response is option B: Problem solving.

Psychoeducation programs serve to 1) educate patients and family members about a particular disorder, 2) teach coping skills and individual and family skills, 3) provide ongoing support to the patient and/or to family members, and 4) offer a problem-solving forum. Not all programs that are designated "psychoeducation" or "family psychoeducation" include all four components listed above. The problem-solving component may be the one least consistently found in psychoeducation programs. **(pp. 305, 307)**

14.4   Which statement is most accurate regarding psychoeducation for PDs?

A. Psychoeducation programs have been developed widely for several of the PDs.
B. Psychoeducation programs for antisocial PD have demonstrated a reduction in violence recidivism.

C. There are some data to suggest psychoeducation is contraindicated for Cluster B disorders.

D. Several studies have shown positive outcomes using psychoeducation in combination with other interventions in avoidant PD.

E. A number of patient and family psychoeducation programs have been developed for Cluster A diagnoses because programs for related Axis I disorders have been successful.

The correct response is option D: Several studies have shown positive outcomes using psychoeducation in combination with other interventions in avoidant PD.

Avoidant PD has several behavioral and theoretical connections to Axis I disorders, and several studies have shown positive outcomes using psychoeducation and graduated exposure techniques, which are the standard psychological interventions used in treating related Axis I disorders such as social phobia. One study (Alden 1989) employing social skills training and patient psychoeducation found significant improvement in most domains. Because the studies aggregate the interventions, it is difficult to parse out the specific effect of psychoeducation. Psychoeducation programs have not been developed widely for PDs with the exception of borderline PD (BPD) (options A, E). Despite the fact that there are many successful programs for related Axis I disorders, no psychoeducation programs have been established for Cluster A problems (option E). There are no data to contraindicate psychoeducation for any PD or cluster of disorders (option C). No studies have specifically evaluated psychoeducation for antisocial PD, although many studies have evaluated various psychoeducation and skills training programs for anger, aggression, or violent behaviors—problems that overlap to some extent with antisocial PD. The extent of this overlap is not clear, however, and the effectiveness of these treatments in reducing violence recidivism is controversial (option B) (Babcock et al. 2004). **(pp. 308–309)**

14.5 In discussion with a patient, it becomes clear her sister has BPD. Which of the following is the best psychoeducational approach to informing the patient about her sister?

A. Suggest that she search the Internet for information on BPD.

B. Describe for her the homogeneous nature of the disorder.

C. Explain how stability across time distinguishes PD from other psychiatric disorders.

D. Note that for BPD we do not yet know what is inherited, what is learned, or how these factors interact.

E. Warn the patient that her sister may have suffered a significant trauma, because trauma is a necessary and sufficient cause of BPD.

The correct response is option D: Note that for BPD we do not yet know what is inherited, what is learned, or how these factors interact.

BPD has a significant level of heritability, with estimates ranging from a low of 15%–20% to a high of 55% (White et al. 2003). It is important to understand that the estimates represent average levels and that for any individual patient the level of heritability could vary considerably. We do not yet know what is inherited, what is learned, or how these factors interact. The Internet is a frequent source of information, a rich resource for useful and accurate psychoeducation, but it includes much that is contradictory and even discredited (option A). Thus clinicians might direct patients and families to specific Web sites such as the Web site for the National Education Alliance for Borderline Personality Disorder (www.borderlinepersonalitydisorder.com). BPD is heterogeneous, with different clusters of problems more prominent in different people (option B).

Whereas stability across time has been used to distinguish PDs from other psychiatric disorders, longitudinal studies have shown them to be only relatively stable (option C). They are more stable than most other disorders, but they do, nonetheless, change, often improving, over time.

The presence of trauma in the history of people who develop BPD is not uncommon (as high as 75% is reported retrospectively in inpatient and outpatient samples; Battle et al. 2004). Trauma has sometimes been hypothesized to be a major cause of BPD, despite data that clearly suggest otherwise. Patients and families should be educated about the fact that trauma is neither necessary nor sufficient to cause BPD (option E). A meta-analysis of its role found only 15% of the variance in BPD's etiology is due to trauma (Fossati et al. 1999). **(pp. 309–311)**

14.6   A colleague asks your thoughts on how to advise her new patient with BPD about treatment options. A psychoeducational approach to informing the patient about treatment should include which of the following?

A. Advise that in terms of evidence-based treatments, mentalization-based therapy has the most supporting studies, with dozens of controlled and uncontrolled trials.
B. Reassure the patient that there are an increasing variety of treatments for BPD and that the vast majority of BPD patients have access to them.
C. Note that it is unreasonable for the patient and her family to have a timetable in mind for recovery.
D. Suggest that if there are no BPD-specific treatments available to the patient, it is more prudent to forgo treatment and instead seek peer support.
E. Inform the patient that there is no medication that is consistently or dramatically helpful in the treatment of BPD.

The correct response is option E: Inform the patient that there is no medication that is consistently or dramatically helpful in the treatment of BPD.

Clinicians need to establish realistic, modest expectations about the benefits from taking medications. This message is important because expectations of benefit are often excessive. Patients with BPD should be told directly that there are no medications that are consistently or dramatically helpful. In terms of evidence-based treatments, although mentalization-based therapy has more recently begun to accumulate substantial support, dialectical behavioral therapy (DBT) has the most supporting studies (option A). Even though an increasing variety of treatments with at least some evidence to support them have been developed for BPD, most of these treatments continue to remain inaccessible to the vast majority of BPD patients (option B). In the absence of available evidence-based treatment or BPD-specific treatments, it may be necessary to identify providers who at least have had experience with treating patients with BPD and who feel comfortable or even enjoy doing so (option D). Patients and families should have a reasonable timetable for change in mind and become active monitors of whether expectable progress is happening (option C). **(pp. 312–313)**

14.7   Which statement most accurately describes the joining phase of Gunderson's multifamily groups for BPD?

A. Relatives from one family join a multifamily group to create an alliance and connection with other families.
B. General information about BPD is provided, but information about family members' history is not elicited.
C. During this phase, acknowledgement of family members' anger and angst is avoided because it undermines the alliance with the patient.
D. The joining phase offers participants the experience of hearing from other families in similar situations.
E. Participants nearing completion of this phase are asked to commit, in general, to a 4-month period for the remainder of this phase of treatment.

The correct response is option E: Participants nearing completion of this phase are asked to commit, in general, to a 4-month period for the remainder of this phase of treatment.

Gunderson's multifamily groups follow a three-phase format: 1) joining, 2) a half-day psychoeducation workshop, and 3) biweekly multifamily group meetings. In the joining phase, the relatives from one family meet alone with the leaders, whose primary goal is to create an alliance and connection with the relatives (option A). Information on the diagnosis of BPD is provided, and history of the family members' experiences and perspectives on their relative's difficulties are shared (option B). Acknowledgement of family members' anger and angst is crucial because it allows for open expression of feelings (option C). Although there is no time limit on this phase of treatment, participants nearing completion of this phase are asked to commit, in general, to a 4-month period for the remainder of this phase. During the second phase of treatment, half-day psychoeducation workshops, participants have the experience of hearing from other families in similar situations (option D). **(pp. 315–316)**

14.8   Which of the following statements does *not* describe DBT-oriented family skills training (DBT-FST)?

A. It offers a forum to put skill acquisition and generalization practice into the family environment.
B. It was developed specifically for family participants, and patients do not attend the sessions.
C. It attempts to educate family participants about BPD.
D. It works to teach a new language of communication based on DBT skills.
E. It promotes an attitude that is nonjudgmental, which is particularly useful for high-stress participant families.

The correct response is option B: It was developed specifically for family participants, and patients do not attend the sessions.

DBT-FST includes both the DBT client and his or her family members. It has four primary goals: 1) to educate family participants about BPD (option C), 2) to teach a new language of communication based on DBT skills (option D), 3) to promote an attitude that is nonjudgmental (option E), and 4) to provide a safe forum in which discussions and problem solving on family issues may occur (option A) so that new communication patterns are established and a new repertoire for problem solving is developed. **(pp. 316–317)**

14.9 In which psychoeducation program does the patient assume the role of co-teacher to inform and educate those people important to him or her?

A. Gunderson's multifamily groups.
B. Systems Training for Emotional Predictability and Problem Solving (STEPPS).
C. Family Connections.
D. DBT- FST.
E. Peer specialist program.

The correct response is option B: Systems Training for Emotional Predictability and Problem Solving (STEPPS).

An essential feature of the STEPPS program is a systems component that encompasses the patient's environment and important individuals in the patient's life with whom he or she has regular contact. The patient assumes the role of co-teacher to inform these individuals about the disorder and also to educate them on skills that are helpful to manage one's emotions more effectively. Family and significant others thus become an integral part of the treatment and are encouraged to attend education and skill sessions to learn ways to support the patient's treatment and to reinforce his or her newly acquired skills. **(p. 318)**

14.10 A 24-year-old woman was recently diagnosed with BPD. Her parents are distressed because the patient refuses to engage in any treatment. The patient's parents feel confused and isolated. What program might be appropriate for the parents?

A. Gunderson's multifamily groups.

B. STEPPS.

C. Family Connections.

D. DBT- FST.

E. Peer specialist program.

The correct response is option C: Family Connections.

Family Connections is a no-cost family education program specifically developed for family members, so patients do not attend. The program was developed to provide all four functions of psychoeducation: education/knowledge, coping and family skills, social support, and problem solving. Family Connections provides the patient's family with an opportunity to develop a support network and learn more about BPD. Patient participation is an important part of Gunderson's multifamily groups, STEPPS, and DBT-FST (options A, B, and D). Peer specialist programs feature peer specialists who offer support to patients (option E). **(p. 318)**

References

Alden L: Short-term structured treatment for avoidant personality disorder. J Consult Clin Psychol 57:756–764, 1989 2600246

Babcock JC, Green CE, Robie C: Does batterers' treatment work? A meta-analytic review of domestic violence treatment. Clin Psychology Rev 23:1023–1053, 2004 14729422

Battle CL, Shea MT, Johnson DM, et al: Childhood maltreatment associated with adult personality disorders: findings from the Collaborative Longitudinal Personality Disorders Study. J Pers Disord 18:193–211, 2004 15176757

Cummings EM, Davies PT, Campbell SB: Developmental Psychopathology and Family Process: Theory, Research, and Clinical Implications. New York, Guilford, 2000

Eisenberg N, Valiente C, Morris AS, et al: Longitudinal relations among parental emotional expressivity, children's regulation, and quality of socioemotional functioning. Dev Psychol 39:3–19, 2003 12518805

Fossati A, Madeddu F, Maffei C: Borderline personality disorders and childhood sexual abuse: a meta-analytic study. J Pers Disord 13:268–280, 1999 10498039

Fruzzetti AE, Shenk C, Hoffman PD: Family interaction and the development of borderline personality disorder: a transactional model. Dev Psychopathol 17:1007–1030, 2005 16613428

White CN, Gunderson JG, Zanarini MC: Family studies of borderline personality disorder: a review. Harv Rev Psychiatry 11:8–19, 2003 12866737

CHAPTER 15

Somatic Treatments

15.1 Which of the following medications has been shown to worsen impulsivity and behavioral dyscontrol in individuals with borderline personality disorder (BPD)?

A. Alprazolam.
B. Fluoxetine.
C. Haloperidol.
D. Lamotrigine.
E. Lithium.

The correct response is option A: Alprazolam.

A study by Cowdry and Gardner (1988) assessed four different medication classes (a first-generation antipsychotic, benzodiazepine, anticonvulsant, and antidepressant) in the treatment of BPD. In this study, alprazolam was associated with no improvement in symptoms and a worsening of impulsivity and dyscontrol. The other medications listed above have all been shown to reduce impulsivity or other symptoms of BPD to some degree. Specifically, fluoxetine (option B) has been shown to improve impulsivity in some studies, haloperidol (option C) has been reported to be superior to placebo across several measures, lamotrigine (option D) has been noted to lead to significant improvement and safety, and lithium (option E) has been reported to reduce impulsive symptoms (although it is associated with a significant potential for morbidity and mortality if taken in overdose, which is a noted risk in this population). **(pp. 328–329)**

15.2 Which of the following medications has been shown to reduce psychoticism in patients with schizotypal PD?

A. Aripiprazole.
B. Clozapine.
C. Quetiapine.
D. Risperidone.
E. Ziprasidone.

The correct response is option D: Risperidone.

Low-dose risperidone has been shown to reduce psychoticism in patients with schizotypal PD. Olanzapine has also been shown to reduce psychoticism in this population. The other antipsychotic medications listed have not been rigorously studied in schizotypal PD. **(pp. 324–325)**

15.3   Which of the following antidepressants has been associated with worsening of symptoms of BPD?

    A. Amitriptyline.
    B. Fluoxetine.
    C. Phenelzine.
    D. Selegiline.
    E. Venlafaxine.

The correct response is option A: Amitriptyline.

Soloff et al. (1986) found that amitriptyline did not perform better than placebo. Amitriptyline was associated with deterioration of behavior in approximately 25% of BPD patients. Other studies have found positive effects for fluoxetine, phenelzine, and venlafaxine (options B, C, E) in treating patients with BPD. Selegiline (option D) has not been studied in this population. **(pp. 323, 327)**

15.4   Which of the following medications has been shown to be helpful in patients with BPD who do not respond to selective serotonin reuptake inhibitors (SSRIs)?

    A. Clonazepam.
    B. Haloperidol.
    C. Lithium.
    D. Omega-3 fatty acids.
    E. Venlafaxine.

The correct response is option E: Venlafaxine.

In a study by Markovitz and Wagner (1995), individuals with BPD who did not respond to an SSRI demonstrated improvement with venlafaxine. Benzodiazepines (clonazepam) (option A) are not recommended in the treatment of BPD. Options B and D have some positive outcomes in this population; however, they have not been specifically studied in patients who did not respond to an SSRI. Lithium (option C) is associated with a significant potential for morbidity and mortality if taken in overdose, which is a noted risk in this population. **(p. 328)**

15.5 Which of the following symptom domains in BPD were improved during treatment with omega-3 fatty acids?

A. Aggression.
B. Anxiety.
C. Impulsivity.
D. Mood lability.
E. Suicidality.

The correct response is option A: Aggression.

In a small double-blind, placebo-controlled trial ($N=30$), omega-3 fatty acids were found to improve aggression and depressive symptoms compared to placebo (Zanarini and Frankenburg 2003). The use of omega-3 fatty acids in the treatment of BPD was further supported in a Cochrane Collaboration Review in 2010 (Stoffers et al. 2010). **(pp. 331, 333)**

15.6 What is the best recommendation for appropriate use of medications in the treatment of BPD?

A. Acute use of medications targeted to specific symptom domains.
B. Acute use of medications to prepare the patient to enter psychotherapy.
C. Avoidance of medications during psychotherapy.
D. Chronic use of medications in patients unable to engage in psychotherapy.
E. Chronic use of medications to reduce overall BPD severity.

The correct response is option A: Acute use of medications targeted to specific symptom domains.

The Cochrane Collaboration Review (Stoffers et al. 2010) noted the importance of identifying clear treatment targets when prescribing medications in BPD and combining medication treatment with psychotherapy. They also recommended discontinuing the medication if there is no improvement in these targets. In a separate meta-analysis of pharmacologic treatment in BPD (Ingenhoven et al. 2010), the authors similarly recommended that medications should be used "to target specific symptom domains." Furthermore, the Australian National Health and Medical Research Council (2012) recently released guidelines that state that "medication should not be used as a primary therapy for BPD," and that "medications should be used in acute crisis situations and discontinued after the crisis is resolved." Thus, the best recommendation is using medications acutely to target specific symptom domains. It would not be appropriate to use medications without psychotherapy (option B), and there is no recommendation for chronic treatment with medications (options D and E). There is also no requirement to avoid medications during psychotherapy (option C). **(pp. 333–334)**

15.7   On the basis of the results of a large meta-analysis of controlled trials, psycho-pharmacologic medications have the largest effect size for treatment of which of the following symptom domains in BPD?

A. Anxiety.
B. Cognitive-perceptual disturbances.
C. Depressed mood.
D. Emptiness.
E. Impulsive-behavioral dyscontrol.

The correct response is option E: Impulsive-behavioral dyscontrol.

Of the symptom domains listed above, impulsive-behavioral dyscontrol has the largest effect size with pharmacologic treatment (specifically, a very large effect size with anticonvulsant mood stabilizers). The effect size is small to large for anxiety (option A) depending on the medication prescribed, small to moderate for depressed mood (option C), and moderate for cognitive-perceptual disturbances (option B). There have been no medications that have been shown to improve emptiness (option D) in BPD. **(pp. 334–335)**

15.8   Which of the following PDs has the strongest evidence base to support the use of psychopharmacologic treatment?

A. Avoidant PD.
B. BPD.
C. Obsessive-compulsive PD.
D. Schizoid PD.
E. Schizotypal PD.

The correct response is option B: BPD.

The evidence base is unfortunately very limited for the pharmacologic treatment of paranoid, schizoid, schizotypal, histrionic, narcissistic, avoidant, and obsessive-compulsive PDs. The greatest evidence exists for the pathophysiology and treatment of BPD. **(pp. 321–322)**

15.9   A 26-year-old patient presents with complaints of mood swings in the context of a recent breakup. She has recently moved and is seeking a new psychiatrist. She states that she has always had problems keeping a relationship for more than a couple of months, noting that the relationship seems "perfect" at first but then suddenly and inexplicably seems to end. She experiences mood swings, intense anger, irritability, and anxiety. She states that she "hates" herself and notes that everyone important in her life has always let her down. She also has a history of making superficial lacerations to her wrists, but she firmly denies any current suicidal thoughts or plans. She is currently taking alprazolam 0.5 mg three times daily, fluoxetine 40 mg daily, and risperidone 2 mg nightly. In addition to active engagement in psychotherapy, which of the following is the most appropriate next step in her treatment?

A. Add valproate.
B. Change fluoxetine to venlafaxine.
C. Increase fluoxetine.
D. Increase risperidone.
E. Taper and discontinue alprazolam.

The correct response is option E: Taper and discontinue alprazolam.

Benzodiazepines have been demonstrated to worsen impulsivity and behavioral dyscontrol. Given this patient's current relationship crisis and increase in her symptoms, the alprazolam should be tapered and discontinued while monitoring for withdrawal. Given the possibility that alprazolam may actually be exacerbating her symptoms, it is important to remove the alprazolam before initiating other medication changes. One could make an argument for adding valproate, changing fluoxetine to venlafaxine, increasing fluoxetine, or increasing risperidone (options A, B, C, D) based on her current symptom domains (see Table 15–1), but these steps should be taken after discontinuing the alprazolam. **(p. 329)**

References

Cowdry RW, Gardner DL: Pharmacotherapy of borderline personality disorder: alprazolam, carbamazepine, trifluoperazine, and tranylcypromine. Arch Gen Psychiatry 45:111–119, 1988 3276280

Ingenhoven T, Lafay P, Rinne T, et al: Effectiveness of pharmacotherapy for severe personality disorders: meta-analyses of randomized controlled trials. J Clin Psychiatry 71:14–25, 2010 19778496

Markovitz PJ, Wagner SC: Venlafaxine in the treatment of borderline personality disorder. Psychopharmacol Bull 31:773–777, 1995 8851652

National Health and Medical Research Council: Clinical Practice Guideline for the Management of Borderline Personality Disorder. Melbourne, Australia, National Health and Medical Research Council, 2012

Soloff PH, George A, Nathan RS, et al: Paradoxical effects of amitriptyline on borderline patients. Am J Psychiatry 143:1603–1605, 1986 3538914

Stoffers JM, Völlm BA, Rücker G, et al: Pharmacological interventions for borderline personality disorder. Cochrane Database of Systematic Reviews 2010, Issue 6. Art. No.: CD005653. DOI: 10.1002/14651858.CD005653.pub2.

Zanarini MC, Frankenburg FR: Omega-3 fatty acid treatment of women with borderline personality disorder: a double-blind, placebo-controlled pilot study. Am J Psychiatry 160:167–169, 2003 12505817

CHAPTER 16

Collaborative Treatment

16.1　What is the best definition of collaborative treatment?

A. A method of delivering cognitive-behavioral therapy (CBT).
B. A treatment relationship that occurs when two or more treatment modalities are provided by more than one mental health or medical professional.
C. A system of care that is only delivered in a particular setting.
D. A treatment that used to be delivered in the primary care setting but has not persisted.

The correct response is option B: A treatment relationship that occurs when two or more treatment modalities are provided by more than one mental health or medical professional.

Collaborative treatment generally occurs when one clinician provides a form of psychotherapy (option A) and another clinician provides psychotropic medication and there is communication between the clinicians. In fact, there may be more than two clinicians, and the setting may vary (options C, D), depending on the type of services delivered. Collaborative treatment is a growing form of care. **(p. 345)**

16.2　*Split treatment* may be viewed as one form of collaborative treatment. How is split treatment different from collaborative care?

A. There is often a lack of communication or agreement between the providers.
B. The bills for care of the patient are split.
C. There is a split in the unconscious and conscious realm of care.
D. The patient realizes that he or she must split his or her time between the hospital and outpatient services.

The correct response is option A: There is often a lack of communication or agreement between the providers.

Although some authors view *split treatment* as a neutral term used to describe division of care among various clinicians, there has been a shift away from using this term. Instead, *collaborative treatment* is now viewed as a favorable term that more accurately encapsulates the way in which providers can work together to further enhance communication and improve patient care. The term *split treatment* has now come to reflect a less ideal situation in which clinicians provide care to the same patient but are not communicating with one another and may not be furthering the patient's overall care. **(pp. 345–346)**

16.3   What is a problem that may occur in split treatment of patients with PDs?

A. Most patients with schizoid traits may ask for increased doses of antidepressants.
B. There are fewer prescriptions for mood stabilizers.
C. Patients with Cluster C traits may become increasingly obsessional.
D. Patients with Cluster B traits tend to split even without a split treatment relationship.

The correct response is option D: Patients with Cluster B traits tend to split even without a split treatment relationship.

Splitting is a defensive process wherein a patient appears to attribute good characteristics almost exclusively to one provider of treatment while attributing to the other treater all the bad or negative feelings. Defensive splitting can be accompanied by *projective identification,* in which the patient projects disavowed aspects of himself or herself onto different treaters. It is important, then, that the treaters not unconsciously identify with these projected characteristics and not feel pressured to respond accordingly. **(p. 346)**

16.4   Why is it important to employ collaborative treatment for patients with PDs?

A. Efficacy studies within this patient population demonstrate superiority of multiple care providers over just one provider.
B. Many patients with PDs often do not respond as well to medications as would patients with other primary diagnoses and thus may need other treatment modalities.
C. Families generally ask for many clinicians to care for their loved one.
D. Strong comparison data show that pharmacotherapy and psychotherapy are only useful in a minority subset of patients with PDs.

The correct response is option B: Many patients with PDs often do not respond as well to medications as would patients with other primary diagnoses and thus may need other treatment modalities.

Many patients with PDs have complex biological and psychosocial issues and may not respond as well to medication as would patients with other primary diagnoses (except perhaps patients with schizotypal PD [Duggan et al. 2008; Herpertz et al. 2007; Koenigsberg et al. 2003; Paris 2003; Soloff 1990, 1998]). Therefore, clinicians often have to provide a combination of pharmacotherapy and psychotherapy, and these may be provided by more than one clinician There are surprisingly few studies, and even fewer randomized, controlled trials, comparing different combinations of treatment modalities to determine the differential efficacy in patients with PDs. While there are studies that compare the use of different pharmacological and non-pharmacological strategies, either alone or in combination, none of them address the use of single versus multiple providers (option A). Families do not generally ask for multiple clinicians. It is too costly, it potentially results in fragmented care, and patients and families appreciate close and trusted doctor-patient relationships (option C). For patients with PDs, no clear conclusions can be drawn concerning the effectiveness of medication versus psychotherapy because there are very few studies that provide strong comparison data. Patients with personality disorders have often been excluded from long-term studies comparing pharmacotherapy, psychotherapy, and combinations (option D). Until more efficacy studies are done with patients with personality disorders, it is important for clinicians to think of using multiple modalities, such as pharmacotherapy and psychotherapy, in the care of patients with PDs. **(pp. 347–348)**

16.5   Patients are increasingly receiving most psychotropic medication prescriptions from which of the following professionals?

A. Cardiologists.
B. Primary care physicians.
C. Psychiatrists.
D. Social workers.

The correct response is option B: Primary care physicians.

Increasingly, collaborative treatment has come to represent a clinical situation in which a primary care physician prescribes psychotropic medication while a nonpsychiatrist clinician, such as a social worker, provides psychotherapy. Social workers do not prescribe medications. More and more psychotropic medications are being prescribed by primary care physicians, rather than psychiatrists. **(p. 345)**

16.6   A managed care company would be most likely to agree with which of the following statements about patients with PDs?

A. They use much less than their share of psychiatric treatment.
B. They use just enough of their share of psychiatric treatment.
C. They should be encouraged to take full advantage of their psychiatric benefit.
D. They use too much or at least more than their share of treatment benefits.

The correct response is option D: They use too much or at least more than their share of treatment benefits.

One of the challenges in caring for patients with PDs and working with utilization reviewers is to convince the reviewers that more than one treatment modality is needed. Because there is often more than one clinician caring for the patient with a PD (collaborative treatment), it is often useful to designate one of the clinicians to report the progress of the treatment and the treatment plan to the reviewer (i.e., have a designated reporter). **(p. 349)**

16.7   Patients with PDs often have mixtures of symptoms and problems, some of which arise from psychosocial issues and others from baseline anxiety, emotional lability, and impulsivity. Which is most likely to occur in the split treatment of a patient with a PD?

A. The psychotherapist may believe that most of the problems arise from psycho-social issues and may be dismissive of the psychopharmacological treatment.
B. The psychopharmacologist may feel that the difficulties are all due to "trait expression" and not prescribe antidepressant medication.
C. The clinicians often call the managed care company to request fewer sessions.
D. Optimally, the psychotherapist will provide pharmacotherapy without discussing this with the psychopharmacologist.

The correct response is option A: The psychotherapist may believe that most of the problems arise from psychosocial issues and may be dismissive of the psychopharmacological treatment.

The increasing use of psychotropic medications in patients with PD fuels the need for the patient to have a clinician who provides pharmacotherapy as well as a clinician who provides psychotherapy. The clinician providing the psychotherapy may feel the medications are not working and thus be dismissive of that component of the treatment. It is important for clinicians to communicate well (option D) in order to understand the full spectrum of relevant psychosocial and biological issues (option B), so that the clinicians do not devalue or undermine the care provided by the other clinician. There are usually not enough visits provided to patients with PD, which is a long-term disorder, so that is extremely rare for clinicians to seek fewer visits for patients with the insurer or managed care company (option C) **(p. 350)**

16.8   Treatment with pharmacotherapy and psychotherapy is a common practice in the treatment of patients with PDs. Match the *factor* with the best *reason.*

Reason		Factor
A. Medications are generally safer and have more tolerable side effects. Safety is particularly important in a subgroup of PD patients, namely, patients with BPD who have very high suicide rates (Healy 2002).	_____ 1.	Managed care plays a significant role.
	_____ 2.	Psychopharmacological agents are in more common use today.
B. Companies are often reluctant to approve treatment sessions for patients with PDs who are not receiving pharmacotherapy.	_____ 3.	Since the 1990s, there are increased types of psychotherapies for patients with PDs.
C. The nature-nurture dichotomy has been replaced by consideration of the subtle interplay of biological predisposition, resulting in traits that are expressed through behavior that is affected by experiential and environmental factors (Rutter, 2002). Such a theory of interaction between biological and psychological factors and life experience supports a multimodal treatment approach (Paris 1994).	_____ 4.	There is a growing appreciation of the role of biological and psychological factors in the etiology of PD symptoms.
D. Treatments such as dialectical behavioral therapy, focused psychotherapy, therapy based on dynamic therapy, interpersonal reconstructive psychotherapy, CBT, and schema-focused CBT.		

Answer key: 1–B; 2–A; 3–D; 4–C.

(p. 354)

The following vignette applies to both questions 16.9 and 16.10:

Mary has been seeing Ms. L, a social worker, for 2 years for trauma she experienced during her military duties and for treatment of BPD. Ms. L sends Mary to see her primary care doctor for medication but does not talk with the doctor ahead of time. When the doctor sees Mary, she believes Mary is getting too dependent on Ms. L. The doctor also surmises that Ms. L is encouraging Mary to leave her current position because of a reenactment of the abuse she felt in the military.

16.9   What might be the best course of action on the part of the primary care doctor?

   A. Request that Mary stop seeing Ms. L.
   B. Request that Mary take an antipsychotic medication.
   C. Call Ms. L, with Mary's permission, and discuss the issues and treatment plan.
   D. Do nothing as Mary's psychotherapy is not a concern for her primary care physician.

The correct response is option C: Call Ms. L, with Mary's permission, and discuss the issues and treatment plan.

Patients with PDs are quite sensitive to disagreements among members of the treatment team (Main 1957; Stanton and Schwartz 1954). It would be best for the clinicians to communicate regarding the biological and psychosocial issues and not to put Mary in the middle. Without talking with Ms. L, it would be premature and inappropriate for the physician to recommend that Mary stop seeing the therapist (option A). There is no evidence from the vignette that an antipsychotic medication would be the optimal first choice (option B). With such a complicated clinical situation, it is be important for Ms. L to communicate with the primary care physician. Each treater should respect what the other is trying to accomplish (option D). **(pp. 356–358)**

16.10 What is a reasonable transference response that Mary might experience upon being referred to the primary care doctor for medication?

   A. Ms. L enjoys caring for Mary.
   B. The psychotherapy with Ms. L is not working.
   C. The primary care doctor is a psychiatrist.
   D. Ms. L is closing her practice.

The correct response is option B: The psychotherapy with Ms. L is not working.

Beginning pharmacotherapy might not be viewed as positive or beneficial to patients, especially those with certain types of PDs. Some patients might feel very negatively toward medication and being sent to another clinician, especially a physician. Patients may feel that their therapists do not like them and are sending them away to someone else to be punished (e.g., receive medication) (option A). Patients may also view referral for psychopharmacology as evidence that the psychotherapy is not working and that another clinician is being brought in because the patient is so bad and difficult. Medication may have positive or negative meaning to the patient, based on past personal or family history of taking medications. Finances are another important aspect to consider before referring patients for psychopharmacology management, because medications and physician fees can be quite expensive. Patients are often reluctant to report such financial burdens. Options C and D would not be considered transference responses. **(p. 359)**

References

Duggan C, Huband N, Smailagic N, et al: The use of pharmacological treatments for people with personality disorder: a systematic review of randomized controlled trials. Personality and Mental Health 2:119–170, 2008

Healy D: The Creation of Psychopharmacology. Cambridge, MA, Harvard University Press, 2002

Herpertz SC, Zanarini M, Schulz CS, et al: World Federation of Societies of Biological Psychiatry (WFSBP) guidelines for biological treatment of personality disorders. World J Biol Psychiatry 8:212–244, 2007 17963189

Koenigsberg HW, Reynolds D, Goodman M, et al: Risperidone in the treatment of schizotypal personality disorder. J Clin Psychiatry 64:628–634, 2003 12823075

Main TF: The ailment. Br J Med Psychol 30:129–145, 1957 13460203

Paris J: Borderline Personality Disorder: A Multidimensional Approach. Washington, DC, American Psychiatric Press, 1994

Paris J: Personality Disorders Over Time: Precursors, Course, and Outcome. Washington, DC, American Psychiatric Publishing, 2003

Rutter M: The interplay of nature, nurture, and developmental influences: the challenge ahead for mental health. Arch Gen Psychiatry 59:996–1000, 2002 12418932

Soloff PH: What's new in personality disorders? An update on pharmacologic treatment. J Pers Disord 4:233–243, 1990

Soloff PH: Algorithms for pharmacological treatment of personality dimensions: symptom-specific treatments for cognitive-perceptual, affective, and impulsive-behavioral dysregulation. Bull Menninger Clin 62:195–214, 1998 9604516

Stanton AH, Schwartz MS: The Mental Hospital: A Study of Institutional Participation in Psychiatric Illness and Treatment. London, Tavistock, 1954

CHAPTER 17

Boundary Issues

17.1 A 34-year-old woman with dependent personality is being treated in psychodynamic psychotherapy by a male therapist. Which of the following therapist actions is most likely to be a boundary violation?

A. Handing her a tissue when she starts to cry.
B. Answering the patient's question about the therapist's marital status.
C. Setting up a brief phone session between appointments.
D. Asking the patient to bring him coffee when she comes for a session.
E. Sending her a postcard while on a prolonged vacation.

The correct response is option D: Asking the patient to bring him coffee when she comes for a session.

It is important to distinguish boundary crossings from boundary violations. *Boundary crossings* are defined as transient, nonexploitative deviations from classical therapeutic or general clinical practice in which the treater steps out to a minor degree from strict verbal psychotherapy. These crossings do not hurt the therapy and may even promote or facilitate it. Examples of this include offering a crying patient a tissue, helping a fallen patient up from the floor, helping an elderly patient to put on a coat, answering selected personal questions, disclosing selected personal information, and writing a patient cards during a long absence (options A, B, E). *Boundary violations,* in contrast, such as the therapist asking the patient to run errands for him, constitute essentially harmful deviations from the normal parameters of treatment—deviations that *do* harm the patient, usually by some sort of exploitation that breaks the rule, "first, do no harm"; usually, it is the therapist's needs that are gratified by taking advantage of the patient in some manner. In the case of violations, the therapy is not advanced and may even be destroyed. Brief, scheduled phone sessions are not harmful deviations from accepted treatment (option C). **(pp. 370–371)**

17.2 When a boundary crossing occurs in therapy, it is essential to first do which of the following?

A. Discuss with the patient at the next available occasion.
B. Apologize to the patient at the next session.
C. Only discuss it if the patient brings it up at the next session.

D. Transfer the patient to another therapist.

E. Emphasize to the patient that this is considered a normal part of therapy.

The correct response is option A: Discuss with the patient at the next available occasion.

An important point about boundary crossings is that when they occur, the therapist should review the matter with the patient on the next available occasion and fully document the rationale, the discussion with the patient, and the description of the patient's response. This advice may be summarized as the "3 Ds": demeanor (remaining professional at all times), debriefing (with the patient at the next session), and documentation (of both the crossing event and its rationale). Under some circumstances, a tactful apology to the patient for misreading a situation may be in order when there is a potential boundary violation (option B), but the subject should first be discussed. It is not recommended that discussion be dependent on the patient bringing up the subject (option C) nor that the patient be transferred or told that boundary crossings are "normal" (options D, E) **(p. 371)**

17.3 A male therapist justifies a sexual relationship with a female patient by stating, "It's not my fault—I was seduced." This is not a valid excuse for which of the following reasons?

A. Financial duty.

B. Power asymmetry.

C. Confidentiality.

D. Context dependence.

E. Setting.

The correct response is option B: Power asymmetry.

Power asymmetry refers to the unequal distribution of power between the two parties in the therapeutic dyad: the therapist has greater social and legal power than the patient. Part of this power derives from the fact that the therapist often has detailed knowledge of the patient, including, theoretically, the patient's weaknesses and vulnerabilities—knowledge that may be used for good or ill. With this power comes the greater responsibility for directing and containing the therapeutic envelope. The occasional plaint, "It's not my fault—the patient seduced me," carries little weight under this formulation. Finances, confidentiality, context, and setting are irrelevant to this issue (options A, C, D, E). **(p. 372)**

17.4 Intrinsic consequences of boundary violations may include which of the following?

A. Ethics complaint to the professional society.

B. Civil lawsuit.

C. Board of registration complaint.

D. Criminal lawsuit.

E. Patient suicide.

The correct response is option E: Patient suicide.

The consequences of boundary problems may be divided into those intrinsic to the therapy and those extrinsic to the therapy. A serious and exploitative boundary violation may doom the therapy and cause the patient to feel (accurately) betrayed and used. The clinical consequences of boundary violations, including sexual misconduct, may encompass the entire spectrum of emotional harms from mild and transient distress to suicide. The extrinsic harms fall into three major categories: civil lawsuits (in some jurisdictions, criminal charges for overtly sexual activity); complaints to the board of registration, the licensing agency; and ethics complaints to the professional society (such as the district branch of the American Psychiatric Association), usually directed to the ethics committee of the relevant organization (options A, B, C, D). **(pp. 372–373)**

17.5 Malpractice insurance will always pay for legal fees involved in which of the following?

A. Any malpractice lawsuit.
B. Any malpractice lawsuit other than for a sexualized boundary violation.
C. Any board of registration complaint other than for a sexualized boundary violation.
D. Ethics complaints.
E. Any board of registration complaint.

The correct response is option B: Any malpractice lawsuit other than for a sexualized boundary violation.

A malpractice suit against the clinician will be defended and—in case of a loss—paid for by the malpractice insurer; however, many insurance policies contain exclusionary language that avoids coverage for the more sexualized forms of boundary violation. A board of registration or licensure complaint is not considered a malpractice issue; therefore, one's insurance policy will often not fund the defense, leaving the doctor with out-of-pocket legal expenses (options C, D, E). **(p. 373)**

17.6 A 39-year-old woman with histrionic personality disorder (PD) tries unsuccessfully to get her therapist to give her a hug. At the end of the session, the therapist walks her to the door and closes it after she leaves. A minute later, the patient starts knocking on the door and loudly calling the therapist's name. An appropriate response might be which of the following?

A. Bringing the patient back into the office and thoroughly discussing her behavior and the reason for acting this way.
B. Telling the patient that if she does not stop this behavior, therapy will need to be terminated.
C. Telling the patient that this behavior is inappropriate and should be discussed at the next session.

D. Bringing the patient back into the office and discussing transfer to another therapist.
E. Calling security to escort the patient out and then calling and referring her to another clinic.

The correct response is option C: Telling the patient that this behavior is inappropriate and should be discussed at the next session.

Dramatic behavior such as this may "trigger" a boundary problem because of the clinician's wish to "turn down the volume." Although patients are free to cross boundaries, the limits must be set by the clinician. This patient above might have been told that the behavior was inappropriate and should be discussed at the next appointment; should the patient refuse to leave, security might be called, and the matter explored at the next session. Difficulty setting boundaries may result from the therapist's countertransference-based inability to deal with his own sadistic feelings about "rejecting" the patient and being able to turn the patient away when she was behaving inappropriately. The therapist should avoid crossing boundaries by prolonging the session (option A) and should also avoid acting on the sadistic impulses by punishing the patient for this behavior (options B, D, E). **(pp. 374–375)**

17.7 A female therapist is treating a 29-year-old man with antisocial PD. The most likely indication that the therapist has committed a boundary violation is which of the following?

A. The patient has started calling the therapist by her first name.
B. The therapist has started the patient on an antidepressant.
C. The therapist has volunteered to testify at a parole hearing for the patient.
D. The patient has developed a maternal transference toward the therapist.
E. The patient is demanding to be placed on alprazolam for anxiety.

The correct response is option C: The therapist has volunteered to testify at a parole hearing for the patient.

From the patient's viewpoint, the boundaries, even if recognized, may be ignored in a goal-directed manner. This may lead to behavior such as calling the therapist by her first name or demanding controlled substances (options A, E). Some common goals of this tendency toward pseudo-closeness are obtaining excusing or exculpatory letters sent to nonclinical recipients; obtaining prescription of inappropriate or inappropriately large amounts of controlled substances; and intervention in the patient's extratherapeutic reality such as testifying at a parole hearing. An unfortunately common clinically observed constellation of boundary problems is the following: a female psychotherapist is treating a male patient with antisocial PD but misses the antisocial elements in the patient, seeing the latter as a needy infant who requires loving care to "get better." In the course of this rescue operation, boundary incursions occur and increase (Gabbard and Lester 2003).

Use of appropriate medication and development of transference do not indicate a boundary violation (options B, D). **(pp. 375–376)**

17.8 Which of the following is defined as the "red flag" that should alert a therapist of an impending boundary violation with a patient who has borderline PD (BPD)?

   A. The therapist's realization that an exception to his or her usual practice is about to be made.
   B. The patient's sense of entitlement and of being "special."
   C. A history of early sexual trauma in the patient.
   D. The therapist's recognition of the patient's unconscious manipulation.
   E. Recognition of "borderline rage" in a patient.

The correct response is option A: The therapist's realization that an exception to his or her usual practice is about to be made.

The patient's sense of entitlement and of being "special" may infect the therapist with the same view of his or her specialness, such that even inappropriate exceptions may be made. However, just noting the sense of entitlement or "borderline rage" or obtaining a history of sexual trauma does not indicate an imminent boundary violation because these are common in many, if not most, patients with BPD (options B, E, C). The surprising power of the manipulation to slip under the clinician's radar, as it were, is one of the more striking findings in the boundary realm. "I sensed that I was doing something that was outside my usual practice and, in fact, outside the pale," the therapist will lament to the consultant, "but somehow I just found myself making an exception with this patient and doing it anyway." Gutheil (1989) described his experience with therapists seeking consultation who would begin their narratives with "I don't ordinarily do this with my patients, but in this case I [insert a broad spectrum of inappropriate behaviors here]." Recognizing the manipulation does not indicate a potential boundary violation (option D). However, a therapist who realizes that an exception to usual practice is about to be made should view this impulse as a red flag signaling the need for reflection and consultation. **(p. 376)**

17.9 Which of the following is the least common cause of boundary transgressions in patients with BPD?

   A. The patient's high suicidal risk.
   B. Countertransference hostility.
   C. The "golden fantasy" entertained by some patients.
   D. Countertransference wish to rescue the patient.
   E. The patient's excessive familiarity and pseudo-closeness with treaters.

The correct response is option E: The patient's excessive familiarity and pseudo-closeness with treaters.

The basic wish to help and heal, unfortunately, may inspire efforts that—no matter how well intended—transgress professional boundaries in problematic ways. The patient's transferential neediness and dependency may evoke a countertransferential need in the therapist to rescue (option D), save, or heal the patient at any cost. Wishes to save the patient from anxiety, depression, or suicide (option A) are common stimuli to boundary violations in the name of rescue. The frustration with patients who do not get better may rise to the level of overt anger, in which the therapist acts out countertransference hostility (option B) by violating boundaries such as confidentiality. Smith (1977) defined the golden fantasy entertained by some patients with BPD (option C) and others; the *golden fantasy* is the belief that all needs—relational, supportive, nurturing, dependent, *and* therapeutic—will be met by the treater. As the patient loses track of what constitutes the therapeutic aspect of the work, the therapist, too, may begin to lose track of the actual parameters within which the treatment should take place. Although patients with BPD may demonstrate excessive familiarity and pseudo-closeness with their therapists, this behavior is more often seen in patients with antisocial PD. **(pp. 375, 378–379)**

17.10 During which of the following times in therapy are boundary issues more likely to emerge in embryonic form?

A. When the patient and therapist first enter the room and the patient sits down.
B. When medication management is discussed.
C. At the beginning of therapy.
D. When the therapy has ended and the patient is moving toward the door.
E. In the middle of the therapy session.

The correct response is option D: When the therapy has ended and the patient is moving toward the door.

Gutheil and Simon (1995) observed that the neutral space and time when both parties rise from their chairs and move toward the door at the end of a session represents an occasion when both parties may feel that the rules do not really apply, because the session is theoretically over. They recommend that therapists pay attention to their experiences and the events and communications occurring during this "window"; a tendency toward crossing or even violating boundaries may emerge in embryonic form during this period, allowing the therapist to open the subject for exploration in the following session and, one hopes, to deflate its problematic nature. Options A, B, C, and E do not appear to be specific to the emergence of potential boundary issues. **(p. 380)**

17.11 If the therapist believes that a boundary crossing may have occurred, what are the next immediate steps?

A. Maintain professional behavior, document, and discharge the patient.
B. Maintain professional behavior, document, and consult with a lawyer.

C. Discuss with the patient, maintain professional behavior, and document.
D. Apologize to the patient, transfer the patient, and document.
E. Discuss with the patient, transfer the patient, and maintain professional behavior.

The correct response is option C: Discuss with the patient, maintain professional behavior, and document.

Any potential boundary excursion of uncertain meaning should be marked by three critical steps: maintenance of professional behavior, discussion with the patient, and documentation. Under some circumstances, a tactful apology to the patient for misreading a situation may also be in order. Failure to perform these steps casts the therapist in the light of one who wants to conceal wrongdoing. Transferring or discharging the patient is not an appropriate initial action (options A, D, E), and although consultation with a lawyer (option B) may eventually be necessary, it is not an immediate step, whereas discussion with the patient is a necessity. **(p. 380)**

References

Gabbard GO, Lester EP: Boundaries and Boundary Violations in Psychoanalysis, 2nd Edition. Washington, DC, American Psychiatric Press, 2003

Gutheil TG: Borderline personality disorder, boundary violations, and patient-therapist sex: medicolegal pitfalls. Am J Psychiatry 146:597–602, 1989 2653055

Gutheil TG, Simon RI: Between the chair and the door: boundary issues in the therapeutic "transition zone." Harv Rev Psychiatry 2:336–340, 1995 9384919

Smith S: The golden fantasy: a regressive reaction to separation anxiety. Int J Psychoanal 58:311–324, 1977 892997

CHAPTER 18

Assessing and Managing Suicide Risk

18.1 In the "acute-on-chronic" risk model for suicidality in personality disorders (PDs), which of the following is considered an acute risk?

A. Childhood sexual abuse.
B. Poor employment history.
C. Multiple prior treaters.
D. Discharge from the hospital.
E. Low socioeconomic status.

The correct response is option D: Discharge from the hospital.

The acute-on-chronic risk assessment model is a clinically relevant tool used to distinguish between nonmodifiable and potentially modifiable risk factors for suicide and suicidal behavior in patients with PDs. Chronic risk factors for suicide relate to those factors which have existed for many months or years such as childhood sexual abuse (option A), poor employment history (option B), multiple prior treaters (option C), or low socioeconomic status (option E). A recent discharge from the hospital is an example of an acute risk or one that has existed for days, weeks, or at most months and can be modified by clinical interventions. **(pp. 386, 398–399)**

18.2 In DSM-5, the diagnostic criteria of recurrent suicidal or self-injurious behaviors are included in which of the following diagnoses?

A. Paranoid PD.
B. All PDs.
C. Antisocial PD.
D. Borderline PD (BPD).
E. Narcissistic PD.

The correct response is option D: Borderline PD (BPD).

PDs are associated with a relatively high prevalence of suicidal behavior and death by suicide. One psychological autopsy study (Schneider et al. 2006) of suicides using semistructured interviews with informants yielded rates of 72.3% of men and 66.7% of women meeting criteria for at least one PD. Another study of completed suicides (Isometsa et al. 1996) concluded that 29.3% of the sample met criteria for at least one PD. Although research evidence supports an association between a number of PD diagnoses and death by suicide, only BPD, the best studied of the PDs, has a diagnostic criterion in the DSM-5 ("recurrent suicidal behavior, gestures, or threats, or self-mutilating behavior") specifically describing suicidal behavior (American Psychiatric Association 2013). DSM-5 diagnostic criteria for paranoid PD, all the PDs, antisocial PD, and narcissistic PD (options A, B, C, E) do not cite suicidality. **(pp. 385, 386–389)**

18.3   What is the estimated lifetime risk of completed suicide for patients with BPD?

A. Substantially less than the other Cluster B PDs.
B. Higher among patients receiving regular outpatient treatment.
C. Between 3% and 10%, depending on the study.
D. About equal to the rate of attempted suicide in BPD.
E. Consistently an 8% rate in all studies.

The correct response is option C: Between 3% and 10%, depending on the study.

The lifetime rate of suicide in individuals with BPD has been estimated to be as high as 10% or as low as 3%, depending on the setting, patient characteristics, and method of study (Paris and Zweig-Frank 2001). The rates of suicide are not consistent (option E) across retrospective and prospective studies and among naturalistic and treatment studies (Paris 2004; Yoshida et al. 2006; Zanarini et al. 2006). The rate of attempted suicide in BPD is much higher than the rate of completed suicide (option D), with estimates of up to 85% having a history of such behavior (Paris 2004), significantly higher than the rate of completed suicide. Studies of patients with BPD receiving treatment (Links et al. 2013; Perry et al. 2009) suggest rates of suicide are lower, not higher, in patients receiving treatment (option B). Psychological autopsy study results (Isometsa et al. 1996) indicated rates of suicide are higher in BPD than in other Cluster B PDs (option A). **(pp. 385, 386–389)**

18.4   Research on suicidality in patients with BPD has indicated the possibility of two patient groups with distinct patterns over time: a group with repeated high-lethality attempts and a group with repeated low-lethality attempts. The group with repeated low-lethality attempts is notable for which of the following?

A. Older age.
B. More psychiatric hospitalizations.
C. Comorbid histrionic or narcissistic PDs.
D. Poor baseline psychosocial functioning.
E. Recruitment for studies from inpatient populations.

The correct response is option C: Comorbid histrionic or narcissistic PDs.

Prospective studies of BPD have demonstrated that the vast majority of patients can expect significant symptom relief over time (Gunderson et al. 2011; Shea et al. 2002, 2009; Zanarini et al. 2012). In an effort to identify the clinical characteristics predicting higher-lethality suicide attempts over time in the subgroup that does not experience symptom relief, one prospective study (Soloff and Chiappetta 2012) identified predictors of continued high-lethality suicide attempts. The low-lethality group was notable for comorbid narcissistic or histrionic PD diagnoses, whereas the high-lethality group was notable for older, not younger, age (option A); more, not fewer, inpatient psychiatric hospitalizations (option B); higher, not lower, baseline functioning (option D); and recruitment from outpatient, not inpatient, samples (option E). **(pp. 392–395)**

18.5   Which of the following is the best description of the stress-diathesis causal model of suicidal behavior?

A. A model suggesting an underlying neurobiologic vulnerability to suicidal behavior in times of stress.
B. Another way to assess and communicate risk of suicide in clinical situations in the acute-on-chronic model.
C. A theory specifically discounting a patient's core personality traits.
D. A model for suicidal behavior developed exclusively for patients with PDs.
E. A model for suicide to be assessed only in retrospective studies.

The correct response is option A: A model suggesting an underlying neurobiologic vulnerability to suicidal behavior in times of stress.

The stress-diathesis causal model of suicidal behavior suggests that specific personality traits may constitute a vulnerability to suicidal behavior at times of stress. The likelihood of suicidal behavior increases when patients experience acute stressors, with a chronic tendency toward pessimism in the case of patients with depression (Mann et al. 1999; Oquendo et al. 2004), as well as in patients with PDs who have personality traits such as emotion dysregulation or impulsive aggression (option D). The stress-diathesis causal model for suicidal behavior should not be confused with the acute-on-chronic risk model, which assists clinicians in assessing and communicating suicidality in patients with PD typically at a chronically elevated suicide risk (option B). The stress-diathesis model suggests that specific personality traits may constitute a vulnerability to suicidal behavior at times of stress, not that those traits should be discounted (option C). Prospective studies of patients with BPD have found that episodes of depression and negative life events predict suicidal behavior at 1 year (Soloff and Chiappetta 2012) and at 3 years (Yen et al. 2005), suggesting that the stress-diathesis model can be studied prospectively (option E). **(pp. 386, 395–396)**

18.6 Crisis management and safety planning for patients with BPD would likely include which of the following?

A. The intervention developed by Stanley and Brown (2012) to facilitate hospitalization of at-risk patients.
B. Use of a variety of interventions with psychotropic medications except for antipsychotics.
C. Avoidance of involvement with family members as part of crisis intervention.
D. Neuroimaging studies.
E. Patient and clinician's collaborative assessment of suicide risk over time.

The correct response is option E: Patient and clinician's collaborative assessment of suicide risk over time.

Collaborative assessment over time including clarification of suicidal thoughts as well as intent would assume patient responsibility in monitoring of risk (Craven et al. 2011). Crisis management and safety planning for patients with BPD can present a challenge even to experienced clinicians when these patients present in a suicidal crisis. There is some evidence that antipsychotic medication may be effective in the treatment of core symptoms of BPD (Vita et al. 2011) and may be useful in reducing patients' anxiety, anger, hostility, and agitation in the emergency department, facilitating assessment, de-escalation of the patient, and development of a treatment plan (option B). The safety planning intervention developed by Stanley and Brown (2012) includes discharge to home from the emergency department and does not necessarily end in inpatient hospitalization (option A). Education of family members about steps to increase safety by restricting access to means of self-injury has been cited as a critical part of crisis management (Links and Hoffman 2005), which would not be possible if family members were not involved in crisis management (option C). Neuroimaging studies have shown promise in defining the structural, metabolic, and functioning biology of brain circuits mediating personality traits such as impulsive aggression and emotion dysregulation in subjects at high risk for suicidal behavior but have not been used for crisis management in this population (option D). **(pp. 395–396, 399–401)**

18.7 Which of the following best describes the changes over time for patients with BPD?

A. Patients with BPD are not likely to show remission of symptoms of the disorder over time.
B. Patients with BPD are likely to show remission of diagnostic criteria for the disorder over time.
C. Patients with BPD will likely have an increased rate of suicide attempts over time.
D. Patients with BPD are more likely to have increasingly impaired social functioning and improved vocational functioning over time.
E. Patients with a history of childhood sexual abuse and BPD will have fewer suicide attempts over time.

The correct response is option B: Patients with BPD are likely to show remission of diagnostic criteria for the disorder over time.

The McLean Study of Adult Development (Zanarini et al. 2012) and the Collaborative Longitudinal Personality Disorders Study (Gunderson et al. 2011; Shea et al. 2002, 2009), which were prospective, longitudinal studies of patients with PDs, reported remission in both symptoms and diagnosis over the course of their follow-ups (option A). Patients with BPD were noted to have progressive remission of diagnostic criteria for the disorder, with acute symptoms, including suicide attempts, remitting most rapidly (option C). A 27-year study of patients hospitalized with BPD (Paris and Zweig-Frank 2001) reported that suicide occurred at an average age of 37 years (option A) and that death by suicide in BPD may occur relatively late in the course of the illness. Only half of the patients with BPD in the McLean Study of Adult Development achieved good social and vocational function by the 10-year follow-up despite symptomatic improvement in 93% of the patients. The patients failing to obtain good psychosocial functioning did so because of impaired vocational achievement not poor social function (option D). In the Collaborative Longitudinal Personality Disorders Study, suicide attempts were predicted by a childhood history of sexual abuse (option E) (Yen et al. 2004). **(pp. 392–394)**

18.8   Health care providers treating suicidal patients with PDs are likely to experience which of the following?

A. Understandable pessimism given data that evidence-based therapies available are not effective in preventing suicidal behavior.
B. Reassurance given the low prevalence of suicidal behavior and death by suicide.
C. Increased concern in cases of recurrent serious suicide attempts.
D. More concern about the risk of suicide for patients with Cluster A or Cluster C disorders than for patients with Cluster B disorder.
E. Optimism when treating patients with antisocial PD given the low rates of suicide in this population.

The correct response is option C: Increased concern in cases of recurrent serious suicide attempts.

Clinicians studying a patient's most serious suicide attempts are able to estimate the severity of a patient's ongoing chronic risk for suicide because the method of previous attempts tends to predict the seriousness of suicide vulnerability (Modai et al. 2004). Recent evidence-based therapies have demonstrated that individual psychotherapy can be effective in preventing future suicide behavior (option A) and in reducing the medical risk of future suicide attempts (McMain et al. 2009). A psychological autopsy study of suicides (Schneider et al. 2006) found that 72.3% of men and 66.7% of women met criteria for at least one PD (option B). Research evidence supports a more clear association between Cluster B

PDs than Cluster A or Cluster C PDA (option D). Patients with antisocial PD are considered to be at elevated risk for suicide (option E). One 5-year study found that 5.7% of subjects died of suicide within the follow-up period (Maddocks 1970), and a Finnish psychological autopsy study of adolescents age 13–19 years found that 17% met criteria for conduct disorder or antisocial PD (Marttunen et al. 1991). **(pp. 385–386, 388–389, 393, 398)**

18.9   What are the findings of studies defining the structural, metabolic, and functional biology of brain circuits mediating personality traits in subjects at high risk for suicidal behavior?

  A. Hippocampal volume gain in structural magnetic resonance imaging (MRI) studies of patients with BPD.
  B. Increased gray matter concentrations of attempters compared with non-attempters in insular cortex.
  C. Improved executive cognitive functioning in borderline subjects under stress leading to suicidal behavior.
  D. Excessive cortical inhibition in functional MRI (fMRI) studies of subjects with BPD.
  E. Hyperarousal of the amygdala and other limbic structures in fMRI studies of subjects with BPD.

The correct response is option E: Hyperarousal of the amygdala and other limbic structures in fMRI studies of subjects with BPD.

Neuroimaging and other studies have begun to define the structural, metabolic, and functional biology of brain circuits that mediate personality traits such as impulsive aggression and emotion dysregulation in subjects at high risk for suicidal behavior. fMRI research has found excessive "bottom-up" activation of the amygdala especially in response to negative emotion (Silbersweig et al. 2007). In structural MRI studies, hippocampal volume loss (option A), with and without diminished volume in the amygdala, is the most widely replicated finding in morphometric studies of BPD (Brambilla et al. 2004; Driessen et al. 2000; Irle et al. 2005; Schmahl et al. 2003; Zetzsche et al. 2007). In a study utilizing voxel-based morphometry (Soloff et al. 2012), attempters of suicide had diminished, not increased, gray-matter concentrations compared to nonattempters in insular cortex (option B), a limbic integration area that is activated in tasks involving social interaction, trust, cooperation, and also social exclusion (rejection). Among patients with BPD, impairment of executive cognitive function under stress, not improvement (option C), has been shown to contribute to suicidal behavior as well as to affective instability and impulsive aggression (Fertuck et al. 2006). fMRI study results suggest that diminished cognitive function during affective arousal may result from the relative failure of "top-down" cortical inhibition from prefrontal and anterior cingulate functions (option D). **(pp. 396–398)**

18.10 Which statistic accurately reflects the prevalence and rates of morbidity and mortality associated with PD diagnoses?

A. The prevalence of PDs from the National Comorbidity Survey Replication of approximately 9% of the general population.
B. An estimation that 5% of psychiatric inpatients meet criteria for BPD.
C. An estimation that 20% of psychiatric outpatients meet criteria for BPD.
D. The estimated lifetime rate of attempted suicide of 25% in patients with BPD.
E. Approximately 36% of men and 33% of women in one psychological autopsy study of completed suicide meeting criteria for at least one PD.

The correct response is option A: The prevalence of PDs from the National Comorbidity Survey Replication of approximately 9% of the general population.

The National Comorbidity Survey Replication estimated the prevalence of PDs to be 9% of the general population (Lenzenweger et al. 2007). The rate of psychiatric inpatients meeting criteria for BPD was noted to be approximately 20%, not 5% (option B) (Lieb et al. 2004). The rate of psychiatric outpatients meeting criteria for BPD was noted to be 10% not 20% (Lieb et al. 2004) (option C). The lifetime estimated rate of attempted suicide in patients with BPD is 85%, not 25% (option D), underscoring the burden of the condition (Paris 2004). Schneider et al. (2006) used a semistructured diagnostic interview in a psychological autopsy study with informants. They found that 72.3% of men and 66.7% of women met criteria for at least one PD (option E). **(pp. 385, 386–388)**

References

American Psychiatric Association: Diagnostic and Statistical Manual of Mental Disorders, 5th Edition. Arlington, VA, American Psychiatric Association, 2013
Brambilla P, Soloff PH, Sala M, et al: Anatomical MRI study of borderline personality disorder patients. Psychiatry Res 131:125–133, 2004 15313519
Craven MA, Links PS, Novak G: Assessment and management of suicide risk, in Psychiatry in Primary Care: A Concise Canadian Pocket Guide. Edited by Goldbloom DS, Davine J. Toronto, ON, Canada, Centre for Addiction and Mental Health, 2011, pp 237–248
Driessen M, Herrmann J, Stahl K, et al: Magnetic resonance imaging volumes of the hippocampus and the amygdala in women with borderline personality disorder and early traumatization. Arch Gen Psychiatry 57:1115–1122, 2000 11115325
Fertuck EA, Lenzenweger MF, Clarkin JF, et al: Executive neurocognition, memory systems and borderline personality disorder. Clin Psychol Rev 26:346–375, 2006 15992977
Gunderson JG, Stout RL, McGlashan TH, et al: Ten-year course of borderline personality disorder: psychopathology and function from the Collaborative Longitudinal Personality Disorders Study. Arch Gen Psychiatry 68:827–837, 2011 21464343
Irle E, Lange C, Sachsse U: Reduced size and abnormal asymmetry of parietal cortex in women with borderline personality disorder. Biol Psychiatry 57:173–182, 2005 15652877
Isometsa ET, Henriksson MM, Heikkinen ME, et al: Suicide among subjects with personality disorders. Am J Psychiatry 153:667–673, 1996 8615412
Lenzenweger MF, Lane MC, Loranger AW, et al: DSM-IV personality disorders in the National Comorbidity Survey Replication. Biol Psychiatry 62:553–564, 2007 17217923
Lieb K, Zanarini MC, Schmahl C, et al: Borderline personality disorder. Lancet 364:453–461, 2004 15288745

Links PS, Hoffman B: Preventing suicidal behaviour in a general hospital service: priorities for programming. Can J Psychiatry 50:490–495, 2005 16127967

Links PS, Kolla NJ, Guimond T, et al: Prospective risk factors for suicide attempts in a treated sample of patients with borderline personality disorder. Can J Psychiatry 58:99–106, 2013 23442897

Maddocks PD: A five year follow-up of untreated psychopaths. Br J Psychiatry 116:511–515, 1970 5449136

Mann JJ, Waternaux C, Haas GL, et al: Toward a clinical model of suicidal behavior in psychiatric patients. Am J Psychiatry 156:181–189, 1999 9989552

Marttunen MJ, Aro HM, Henriksson MM, et al: Mental disorders in adolescent suicide: DSM-III-R axes I and II diagnoses in suicides among 13- to 19-year-olds in Finland. Arch Gen Psychiatry 48:834– 839, 1991 1929774

McMain SF, Links PS, Gnam WH, et al: A randomized trial of dialectical behavior therapy versus general psychiatric management for borderline personality disorder. Am J Psychiatry 166:1365–1374, 2009 19755574

Modai I, Kuperman J, Goldberg I, et al: Suicide risk factors and suicide vulnerability in various psychiatric disorders. Med Inform Internet Med 29:65–74, 2004 15204611

Oquendo MA, Galfalvy H, Russo S, et al: Prospective study of clinical predictors of suicidal acts after a major depressive episode in patients with major depressive disorder or bipolar disorder. Am J Psychiatry 161:1433–1441, 2004 15285970

Paris J: Half in love with easeful death: the meaning of chronic suicidality in borderline personality disorder. Harv Rev Psychiatry 12:42–48, 2004 14965853

Paris J, Zweig-Frank H: A 27-year follow-up of patients with borderline personality disorder. Compr Psychiatry 42:482–487, 2001 11704940

Perry JC, Fowler JC, Bailey A, et al: Improvement and recovery from suicidal and self-destructive phenomena in treatment-refractory disorders. J Nerv Ment Dis 197:28–34, 2009 19155807

Schmahl CG, Vermetten E, Elzinga BM, et al: Magnetic resonance imaging of hippocampal and amygdala volume in women with childhood abuse and borderline personality disorder. Psychiatry Res 122:193–198, 2003 12694893

Schneider B, Wetterling T, Sargk D, et al: Axis I disorders and personality disorders as risk factors for suicide. Eur Arch Psychiatry Clin Neurosci 256:17–27, 2006 16133739

Shea MT, Stout R, Gunderson J, et al: Short-term diagnostic stability of schizotypal, borderline, avoidant, and obsessive-compulsive personality disorders. Am J Psychiatry 159:2036–2041, 2002 12450953

Shea MT, Edelen MO, Pinto A, et al: Improvement in borderline personality disorder in relation to age. Acta Psychiatr Scand 119:143–148, 2009 18851719

Silbersweig D, Clarkin JF, Goldstein M, et al: Failure of fronto-limbic inhibitory function in the context of negative emotion in borderline personality disorder. Am J Psychiatry 164:1832–1841, 2007 18056238

Soloff PH, Chiappetta L: Prospective predictors of suicidal behavior in borderline personality disorder at 6-year follow-up. Am J Psychiatry 169:484–490, 2012 22549208

Soloff PH, Pruitt P, Sharma M, et al: Structural brain abnormalities and suicidal behavior in borderline personality disorder. J Psychiatr Res 46:516–525, 2012 22336640

Stanley B, Brown GK: Safety planning intervention: a brief intervention to mitigate suicide risk. Cogn Behav Pract 19:256–264, 2012

Vita A, De Peri L, Sacchetti E: Antipsychotics, antidepressants, anticonvulsants, and placebo on the symptom dimensions of borderline personality disorder. J Clin Psychopharmacol 31:613–624, 2011 21869691

Yen S, Shea MT, Sanislow CA, et al: Borderline personality disorder criteria associated with prospectively observed suicidal behavior. Am J Psychiatry 161:1296–1298, 2004 15229066

Yen S, Pagano ME, Shea MT, et al: Recent life events preceding suicide attempts in a personality disorder sample: findings from the Collaborative Longitudinal Personality Disorders Study. J Consult Clin Psychol 73:99–105, 2005 15709836

Yoshida K, Tonai E, Nagai H, et al: Long-term follow-up study of borderline patients in Japan: a preliminary study. Compr Psychiatry 47:426–432, 2006 16905408

Zanarini MC, Frankenburg FR, Hennen J, et al: Prediction of the 10-year course of borderline personality disorder. Am J Psychiatry 163:827–832, 2006 16648323

Zanarini MC, Frankenburg FR, Reich DB, et al: Attainment and stability of sustained symptomatic remission and recovery among patients with borderline personality disorder and axis II comparison subjects: a 16-year prospective follow-up study. Am J Psychiatry 169:476–483, 2012 22737693

Zetzsche T, Preuss UW, Frodl T, et al: Hippocampal volume reduction and history of aggressive behavior in patients with borderline personality disorder. Psychiatry Res 154:157–170, 2007 17306512

CHAPTER 19

Substance Use Disorders

19.1 What is the estimated prevalence of alcohol use disorders in patients with DSM-IV personality disorders (PDs)?

A. 10%.
B. 20%.
C. 30%.
D. 40%.
E. 50%.

The correct response is option D: 40%.

In a clinical sample of nearly 700 individuals with DSM-IV PDs, the prevalence of alcohol use disorders was 40.9% (McGlashan et al. 2000). **(p. 408)**

19.2 What is the estimated prevalence of drug use disorders in patients with DSM-IV PDs?

A. 10%.
B. 20%.
C. 30%.
D. 40%.
E. 50%.

The correct response is option D: 40%.

In a clinical sample of nearly 700 individuals with DSM-IV PDs, the prevalence of drug use disorders was 37.3%. **(p. 408)**

19.3 Which of the following PDs is classified as an "externalizing disorder"?

A. Avoidant.
B. Schizotypal.
C. Antisocial.
D. Schizoid.
E. Paranoid.

The correct response is option C: Antisocial.

In the exploration of the epidemiology of PDs, there is substantial evidence for a "metastructure" of psychopathology, distinguishing between "internalizing" and "externalizing" disorders. Externalizing disorders include antisocial PD and substance use disorders, whereas avoidant, schizotypal, schizoid, and paranoid PDs may be components of a "thought disorder" subdimension of the "internalizing" dimension (options A, B, D, E) (Keyes et al. 2013). Borderline PD (BPD), in contrast, may straddle the internalizing and externalizing dimensions (Eaton et al. 2011). **(p. 409)**

19.4   On what should the treatment focus during the initial phase of psychotherapy with a patient with a dual diagnosis of PD and substance use disorder?

A. Confronting and challenging maladaptive traits.
B. Cognitive-affective processes.
C. Transference/countertransference.
D. Establishment and maintenance of abstinence.
E. Interpersonal relationships.

The correct response is option D: Establishment and maintenance of abstinence.

During the earlier sessions, it is often best to place the greatest emphasis on the establishment and maintenance of abstinence but with a secondary focus on identification of and psychoeducation about maladaptive personality traits. During later sessions, once a strong therapeutic relationship is established and substance-related concerns have become less pressing, a greater emphasis can be placed on confronting and changing maladaptive traits, cognitive-affective processes, or interpersonal relationships, including the relationship with the therapist (transference/countertransference) (options A, B, C, E). **(p. 419)**

19.5   Which of the following types of treatment is most useful in patients with dual diagnosis of substance use disorder and PD?

A. Dialectical behavioral therapy.
B. Cognitive-behavioral therapy.
C. Psychodynamic psychotherapy.
D. Motivational interviewing.
E. Supportive psychotherapy plus Alcoholics Anonymous.

The correct response is option E: Supportive psychotherapy plus Alcoholics Anonymous.

Psychotherapy with patients who have both substance use disorder and PD is often insufficient as a stand-alone treatment (options A, B, C, D). Psychotherapy is likely to be most useful if it is offered as part of a comprehensive program incorporating varied treatment modalities (individual and group therapy, pharmaco-therapy if needed) and external resources (e.g., Alcoholics Anonymous or Narcotics Anonymous meetings, residential treatment, detoxification, metha-done maintenance program). **(p. 419)**

19.6 Which of the following pharmacotherapies is generally contraindicated in pa-tients with comorbid PDs and substance abuse disorders?

A. Neuroleptics.
B. Benzodiazepines.
C. Selective serotonin reuptake inhibitors (SSRIs).
D. Lithium.
E. Buspirone.

The correct response is option B: Benzodiazepines.

Benzodiazepines are generally contraindicated for this group because of the risk of addiction and of paradoxical reactions involving behavioral disinhibition (Cowdry and Gardner 1988). Neuroleptics, SSRIs, lithium, and buspirone all have varying indications in treating patients with substance use disorders and do not carry a general contraindication. **(p. 420)**

19.7 The causal pathway explaining the high comorbidity between substance use dis-orders and PDs, which suggests that PDs *contribute* to the development of sub-stance use, is known as which of the following?

A. The behavioral disinhibition pathway.
B. The stress reduction pathway.
C. The reward sensitivity pathway.
D. The primary PD model.
E. The common factor model.

The correct response is option D: The primary PD model.

Given the high comorbidity between substance use and PD, it is reasonable to speculate that the syndromes are in some way causally linked. The behavioral disinhibition pathway (option A) predicts that individuals with antisocial and impulsive traits have lower thresholds for behaviors such as alcohol and drug abuse. The stress reduction pathway (option B) regards substance use as self-medication for the anxiety and mood instability that individuals with PDs my ex-hibit in response to stressful life events. The reward sensitivity pathway (option C) regards the positive, reinforcing properties of substance use as the motivating factor among individuals scoring high on traits such as novelty seeking, reward seeking, extraversion, and gregariousness. The common factor model (option E) holds that both personality and substance use disorder have an independent, common cause consistent with a psychobiological model that they are genetically or biologically related. The primary PD model is correct; it suggests that pathological personality traits contribute to the development of substance use disorders. **(pp. 411–413)**

19.8   Which of the following PDs when comorbid with a substance use disorder predicts the best outcome with a modified version of DBT, known as DBT-S?

A. Borderline.
B. Antisocial.
C. Obsessive-compulsive.
D. Narcissistic.
E. Schizotypal.

The correct response is option A: Borderline.

Overall, studies indicate support for DBT-S among patients with BPD and comorbid substance use disorder. However, DBT-S has not been studied for other PDs. Encouraging results from patients with BPD should not be extrapolated to other PDs, especially because antisocial PD has been described as a possible contraindication for DBT (Linehan and Korslund 2006). **(p. 417)**

19.9   Which of the following best describes the difference between DSM-IV and DSM-5 when describing substance abuse versus dependence?

A. In DSM-IV, substance abuse and substance dependence are a single disorder.
B. In DSM-5, substance abuse and substance dependence are a single disorder.
C. In DSM-IV, the presence of tolerance and withdrawal are not criteria that differentiate substance dependence from substance abuse.
D. In DSM-5, the presence of tolerance and withdrawal are criteria that did not differentiate substance dependence from substance abuse.
E. There are no differences in the DSM-IV and DSM-5 criteria for substance abuse and substance dependence.

The correct response is option B: In DSM-5, substance abuse and substance dependence are a single disorder.

DSM-IV used a system consisting of two types of substance use disorder: abuse and dependence (option A). This was problematic because abuse had inconsistent reliability and validity, whereas dependence was consistently shown to be reliable and valid (Hasin et al. 2006). In DSM-5, the definitions of substance use disorders have changed, with abuse and dependence replaced by a single substance use disorder (Hasin et al. 2013). This disorder is defined by 11 criteria: all seven of the DSM-IV dependence criteria, three of the four DSM-IV abuse criteria (legal problems as a criterion was dropped), and craving. DSM-IV includes tolerance and withdrawal as two of the seven dependence criteria, whereas DSM-5 includes tolerance and withdrawal as criteria for the new substance use disorder (option E). DSM-5 does not differentiate between substance abuse and substance dependence (options C and D). **(p. 421)**

19.10   Which of the following PDs is *not* more prevalent among patients with substance use disorders?

A. Borderline.
B. Antisocial.
C. Obsessive-compulsive.
D. Narcissistic.
E. Schizotypal.

The correct response is option C: Obsessive-compulsive.

The most common PDs in the general population (among individuals without co-occurring substance use disorders) are obsessive-compulsive PD (7.9%), paranoid PD (4.4%), antisocial PD (3.6%), schizoid PD (3.1%), avoidant PD (2.4%), histrionic PD (1.8%), and dependent PD (0.5%) (Grant et al. 2005). Among individuals with 12-month substance use disorders, 8.2% had lifetime schizotypal PD (option E) (Pulay et al. 2009), 14.1% had lifetime BPD (option A) (Grant et al. 2008), and 11.8% had narcissistic PD (option D) (Stinson et al. 2008). The prevalence of antisocial PD among respondents with lifetime drug use disorders was 18.3% (option B) (Goldstein et al. 2007). See Table 19–1 provided below. **(pp. 408–409)**

Summary of NESARC findings on the prevalence and odds ratios of substance use disorders and personality disorders

	Prevalence (%)		OR of lifetime PD and:		
	PD among SUD	SUD among PD	12-month SUD	12-month AUD	12-month DUD
Antisocial[a]	18.3 (DUD)	—	—	8.0	11.3
Borderline[b]	14.1	50.7	3.4	2.7	5.6
Narcissistic[b]	11.8	40.6	2.4	2.2	3.7
Schizotypal[b]	5.9	44.1	2.5	2.0	4.7

Note.   AUD=alcohol use disorder; DUD=drug use disorder; NESARC=National Epidemiologic Survey on Alcohol and Related Conditions; OR=odds ratio; PD=personality disorder; SUD=substance use disorder.
[a]ORs significant at $\alpha=0.05$.
[b]ORs significant at $\alpha=0.01$, and adjustment made for sociodemographic characteristics.
Source.   Data from NESARC studies as described in text.

References

Cowdry RW, Gardner DL: Pharmacotherapy of borderline personality disorder: alprazolam, carbamazepine, trifluoperazine, and tranylcypromine. Arch Gen Psychiatry 45:111–119, 1988 3276280
Eaton NR, Krueger RF, Keyes KM, et al: Borderline personality disorder comorbidity: relationship to the internalizing-externalizing structure of common mental disorders. Psychol Med 41:1041–1050, 2011 20836905
Goldstein RB, Compton WM, Pulay AJ, et al: Antisocial behavioral syndromes and DSM-IV drug use disorders in the United States: results from the National Epidemiologic Survey on Alcohol and Related Conditions. Drug Alcohol Depend 90:145–158, 2007 17433571

Grant BF, Stinson FS, Dawson DA, et al: Co-occurrence of DSM-IV personality disorders in the United States: results from the National Epidemiologic Survey on Alcohol and Related Conditions. Compr Psychiatry 46:1–5, 2005 15714187

Grant BF, Chou SP, Goldstein RB, et al: Prevalence, correlates, disability, and comorbidity of DSM-IV borderline personality disorder: results from the wave 2 National Epidemiologic Survey on Alcohol and Related Conditions. J Clin Psychiatry 69:533–545, 2008 18426259

Hasin D, Hatzenbuehler ML, Keyes K, et al: Substance use disorders: Diagnostic and Statistical Manual of Mental Disorders, fourth edition (DSM-IV) and International Classification of Diseases, tenth edition (ICD-10). Addiction 101 (suppl 1):59–75, 2006 16930162

Hasin D, O'Brien CP, Auriacombe M, et al: DSM-5 criteria for substance use disorders: recommendations and rationale. Am J Psychiatry 170:834–851, 2013 23903334

Keyes KM, Eaton NR, Krueger RF, et al: Thought disorder in the meta-structure of psychopathology. Psychol Med 43:1673–1683, 2013 23171498

Linehan MM, Korslund KE: Dialectical behavior therapy: from soup to nuts. Workshop presentation at the annual meeting of the Association for Behavioral and Cognitive Therapies. Chicago, IL, November 15–16, 2006

McGlashan TH, Grilo CM, Skodol AE, et al: The Collaborative Longitudinal Personality Disorders Study: baseline Axis I/II and II/II diagnostic co-occurrence. Acta Psychiatr Scand 102:256–264, 2000 11089725

Pulay AJ, Stinson FS, Dawson DA, et al: Prevalence, correlates, disability, and comorbidity of DSM-IV schizotypal personality disorder: results from the wave 2 national epidemiologic survey on alcohol and related conditions. Prim Care Companion J Clin Psychiatry 11:53–67, 2009 19617934

Stinson FS, Dawson DA, Goldstein RB, et al: Prevalence, correlates, disability, and comorbidity of DSM-IV narcissistic personality disorder: results from the wave 2 national epidemiologic survey on alcohol and related conditions. J Clin Psychiatry 69:1033–1045, 2008 18557663

CHAPTER 20

Antisocial Personality Disorder and Other Antisocial Behavior

20.1   What do epidemiologic studies reveal about women with antisocial personality disorder (ASPD)?

A. Those who have children have fewer children than do non-antisocial women.
B. They engage in more sexual misbehavior than do their male counterparts.
C. They are as likely as boys to have engaged in fighting, use of weapons, cruelty to animals, or setting fires.
D. Women and men have an equal prevalence of ASPD.
E. They marry at an older age than do their non-antisocial peers.

The correct response is option B: They engage in more sexual misbehavior than do their male counterparts.

Robins (1966) observed that troubled girls who were later diagnosed as antisocial were more likely than boys to have engaged in sexual misbehavior and had a later onset of behavioral problems. As women, they married at a younger age than their non-antisocial peers (option E). Women who had ASPD and had children had more of them than non-antisocial women (option A). Other data on gender differences suggest that antisocial boys are more likely than antisocial girls to engage in fighting, use weapons, engage in cruelty to animals, or set fires (option C). The higher prevalence of ASPD in men has been questioned, yet clinical and epidemiological data are consistent in showing a male preponderance (option D). **(pp. 437–438)**

20.2   What are common attributes of people with ASPD?

A. They generally show remorse after involvement in negative activity.
B. They fail to learn from the negative results of their behavior.
C. They show typical empathy for those negatively affected by their behavior.

212

D. They often manifest micropsychotic episodes.

E. Their symptomatology rarely presents before age 18 years.

The correct response is option B: They fail to learn from the negative results of their behavior.

Attributes of ASPD include a lack of empathy for others (option C) and rare experiences of remorse (option A), in addition to failure to learn from the negative results of their behavior. Although there is no epidemiologic evidence of an increased incidence of mania, psychoses or bipolar disorder can also lead to violent or assaultive behavior and should be considered (i.e., ruled out, not comorbid) as a cause of antisocial behavior (option D). Although the requirement for an earlier conduct disorder diagnosis has been removed in DSM-5, epidemiologic data support that among the few variables predictive of long-term adjustment the variety and severity of childhood behavioral problems were the best predictors of adult antisocial outcome (option E) (Robins 1966). **(pp. 429, 434, 444)**

20.3 What does epidemiologic evidence reveal about children with conduct disorder?

A. The prevalence of conduct disorder is evenly distributed between boys and girls.

B. An estimated 50% of girls eventually develop ASPD.

C. An estimated 75% of boys eventually develop ASPD.

D. By age 11 years, 80% of future cases have had a first symptom.

E. The disorder affects approximately 45% of children in the general population.

The correct response is option D: By age 11 years, 80% of future cases have had a first symptom.

Conduct disorder is a predominantly male disorder (option A) and affects approximately 5%–15% of children (option E) (Black 2013). The disorder has an early onset and is generally present by the preschool years, usually by age 8. By age 11, 80% of future cases have had a first symptom (Robins and Price 1991). Most children with conduct disorder do not develop adult ASPD, but they remain at high risk, with an estimated 25% of girls (option B) and 40% of boys (option C) eventually developing ASPD (Robins 1987). **(p. 434)**

20.4 What differences between men and women did the National Epidemiologic Survey on Alcohol and Related Conditions (NESARC) study of antisocial personality symptoms show?

A. Men were more likely than women to be deceitful.

B. Men were more likely than women to be impulsive and fail to plan ahead.

C. Men were more likely than women to consistently be irresponsible.

D. Men were more likely than women to lack remorse for their harmful actions.

E. Men were more likely than women to be reckless.

The correct response is option E: Men were more likely than women to be reckless.

In the study, men were more likely to be reckless and to reoffend. They demonstrated roughly the same tendency as women to demonstrate irritability, aggressiveness, and feeling no remorse (option D). The females in the study were more likely to have symptoms of deceitfulness, impulsivity, and irresponsibility (options A, B, C). See Table 20–2 provided below. **(pp. 437–438)**

Antisocial personality disorder (ASPD) symptoms in 305 women and 750 men in the NESARC study

Symptoms	Women	Men	Total
Repeated unlawful behaviors, %	81	85	84
Deceitfulness, %	56	46	49
Impulsivity/failure to plan ahead, %	62	54	56
Irritability/aggressiveness, %	74	75	75
Recklessness, %	62	85	79
Consistent irresponsibility, %	89	86	87
Lack of remorse, %	53	52	52
Total ASPD criteria since age 15, mean	4.8	4.8	4.8
Lifetime violent symptoms, mean	3.0	3.3	3.2

Note. NESARC=National Epidemiologic Survey on Alcohol and Related Conditions.
Source. Adapted from Goldstein et al. 2007.

20.5 Which mainstay pharmacologic treatment appears to be the most effective and well supported in the literature when treating ASPD?

A. Risperidone 0.5–2 mg qd.
B. Naltrexone 50 mg qd.
C. Lamotrigine 100–200 mg qd.
D. Clonazepam 0.5–1.5 mg bid.
E. Treatment, if offered, is targeted to any associated mood-substance-related issues.

The correct response is option E: Treatment, if offered, is targeted to any associated mood-substance-related issues.

No drugs are routinely used for the treatment of ASPD, and none are approved by the U.S. Food and Drug Administration. Medications are sometimes used "off-label" to treat antisocial persons, generally for aggressive behaviors and irritability or co-occurring disorders. The use of psychotropic medications to treat ASPD was reviewed by the National Collaborating Centre for Mental Health (2009), commissioned by the National Institute for Health and Clinical Excellence in the United Kingdom. The review was unable to identify any randomized controlled trials conducted in persons with ASPD. The report concluded that the sparse evidence did not support the routine use of medication for antisocial persons, but medication for co-occurring disorders should be used according to guidelines for the disorder in question (e.g., major depression). **(p. 445)**

20.6 Which of the following correctly describes ASPD?

A. Misbehaviors seen in ASPD tend to improve with age.
B. Married individuals with ASPD are more symptomatic than those that are unmarried.
C. ASPD has not been linked to an increased risk for mood disorder.
D. ASPD is not associated with an increased risk of substance abuse.
E. As the etiology of ASPD is biochemical, family factors play little role in the development of ASPD.

The correct response is option A: The misbehaviors seen in ASPD tend to improve with age.

The work of Robins (1966) and Black et al. (1995a, 1995b) shows that most dangerous and destructive behaviors associated with ASPD may improve or remit; however, other troublesome problems remain. Older people with ASPD are less likely to commit crimes or become violent, although many remain troublesome to their families and the community. Some fail to improve at all. When improvement occurs, it typically follows many years of antisocial behavior that has stunted the individual's educational and work achievement, thus limiting their potential achievement. Marriage (option B) is another moderating variable. In Robins' (1966) study more than half of married antisocial persons improved, but few unmarried persons did so. Recently, Burt et al. (2010) used twin data to show that men with lower levels of antisocial behavior were more likely to marry, and those who married engaged in less antisocial behavior than their unmarried co-twin. These data appear to confirm Robins's observation that marriage has a buffering effect on antisocial behavior, and the data are largely consistent with those of S. and E. Glueck (Sampson and Laub 1993), whose work linked job stability and marital attachment with improvement. ASPD is associated with high rates of substance misuse, mood and anxiety disorders (option C), attention-deficit/hyperactivity disorder (ADHD), pathological gambling, and other PDs (e.g., borderline personality disorder [BPD]) (Black 2013; Ullrich and Coid 2009). In the NESARC study, the odds ratio for a lifetime alcohol use disorder in antisocial persons was nearly 8 times expected, and the risk for a lifetime drug use disorder was over 11 times expected (option D) (Compton et al. 2005). Patterns of association of adult antisocial behavior with co-occurring substance use disorders are similar but more modest than those with ASPD (Goldstein et al. 2007). Child abuse is reported to contribute to the development of ASPD. Parents of persons who develop ASPD are often incompetent, absent, or abusive (Robins 1966, 1987) (option E). **(pp. 436, 440, 441–442)**

20.7 Which of the following is thought to be a risk factor for the development of ASPD?

A. Low rates (2%–4%) of electroencephalographic abnormalities.
B. Possessing a high-activity variant of the MAOA gene.
C. Having antisocial siblings.
D. As children, being cared for by multiple caretakers.
E. An increased volume of prefrontal gray matter.

The correct response is option C: Having antisocial siblings.

Research supports a genetic diathesis for antisocial behavior. The evidence from more than 100 family, twin, and adoption studies shows that antisocial behavior runs in families in part because of the transmission of genes (Slutske 2001). In fact, nearly 20% of first-degree relatives of antisocial persons will have ASPD themselves (Guze et al. 1967). A review of twin study data showed monozygotic concordance of nearly 67% compared with 31% concordance for dizygotic twins (Brennan and Mednick 1993). Adoption studies have shown that ASPD is more frequent in adoptees with antisocial biologic relatives (Cadoret et al. 1985). The presence of electroencephalographic abnormalities in nearly half of antisocial persons (option A), along with high rates of minor facial anomalies, learning disorders, enuresis, and behavioral hyperactivity further suggests that ASPD is a neurodevelopmental syndrome. Although childhood abuse is also a known correlate, there are no data to support a relationship to multiple nonabusive caregivers (option D). An important study in the new era of molecular genetics points to the influence of the monoamine oxidase A gene, MAOA. (Monoamine oxidase is an enzyme that breaks down the neurotransmitter serotonin.) The low-activity variant of the gene has been found in antisocial persons who were severely abused as children (Caspi et al. 2002). In contrast, children who had a high-activity variant of the gene rarely became antisocial, despite the presence of abuse (option B). In regard to magnetic resonance imaging data, Raine et al. (2000) reported that antisocial men had reduced gray matter volume in the prefrontal lobes (option E). This was the first indication that anomalies in these structures may underlie some antisocial behavior (Raine et al. 2000). In an attempt to localize symptoms, they looked at a group of pathological liars—a common symptom in ASPD (Yang et al. 2007). The liars had an *increase* in prefrontal white matter volume, prompting them to compare this finding with "Pinocchio's nose" (i.e., repeated lying activates the prefrontal circuitry leading to permanent changes in brain structure). More recently, they found smaller amygdalae in psychopathic individuals compared with control subjects, possibly explaining the shallow emotions observed in psychopathic persons (Yang et al. 2009). **(pp. 438–440)**

20.8 What abnormal pathophysiology is associated with ASPD?

A. Low cortisol levels.
B. High testosterone levels.
C. An elevated startle response.

D. Smaller ventricles on neuroimaging.

E. A low resting pulse rate and low skin conductance.

The correct response is option E: A low resting pulse rate and low skin conductance.

Autonomic hypoarousal (option C) has been posited as underlying psychopathy, a condition that likely constitutes a poor-prognosis subset of those with ASPD (Hare 1986). Psychopathic persons require greater sensory input to produce normal brain functioning than normal subjects, possibly leading these individuals to seek potentially dangerous or risky situations to raise their level of arousal to desired levels. Evidence supporting this theory includes the finding that antisocial adults (and youth with conduct disorder) have low resting pulse rates, low skin conductance, and increased amplitude on event-related potentials (Scarpa and Raine 1997). There are no data to support abnormal cortisol, testosterone, or ventricular size as associations with ASPD (options A, B, D). **(pp. 438–439)**

20.9 Which of the following should be included in the differential diagnosis of ASPD?

A. BPD.

B. Obsessive-compulsive disorder.

C. Generalized anxiety disorder.

D. Pervasive developmental disorder.

E. Complicated grief.

The correct response is option A: BPD.

The differential diagnosis of ASPD includes other PDs (e.g., BPD), substance use disorders, psychotic and mood disorders, intermittent explosive disorder, and medical conditions such as temporal lobe epilepsy (Black 2013). Options B, C, D, and E are not listed as part of a differential diagnosis of ASPD. **(pp. 443–444)**

20.10 Which of the following is difficult to distinguish from conduct disorder in the evaluation of a child?

A. Oppositional defiant disorder.

B. Posttraumatic stress disorder.

C. Normal development.

D. Adjustment disorder with mixed emotional features.

E. Separation anxiety disorder.

The correct response is option A: Oppositional defiant disorder.

The differential diagnosis in children with conduct disorder includes oppositional defiant disorder, ADHD, autistic spectrum disorder, and psychotic and mood disorders, all of which can be associated with sporadic verbal outbursts or physical assaults. Arguably, the most difficult aspect of diagnosis involves distinguishing between conduct disorder and oppositional defiant disorder. The child with oppositional defiant disorder is difficult and uncooperative, but his or her behavior generally does not involve outright aggression, destruction of property, theft, or deceit, as with conduct disorder. A child with ADHD may be inattentive, hyperactive, or disruptive but usually does not violate the rights of others or societal norms. Both ASPD and conduct disorder are distinguishable from normal behavior (option C). Most children experience episodes of rambunctious behavior that can be accompanied by inappropriate language or destructive acts. Similarly, many children or adolescents engage in reckless behavior, vandalism, or even minor criminal activity such as shoplifting, often involving peers. Isolated acts of misbehavior are inconsistent with the diagnosis of either conduct disorder or ASPD, which involve repetitive misbehavior over time. Options B, D, and E are not listed as part of a differential diagnosis. **(pp. 443–444)**

20.11 What is the most well studied and effective mode of psychotherapy in ASPD?

A. Psychoanalysis.
B. Group therapy.
C. Interpersonal therapy.
D. Applied behavioral analysis.
E. There are insufficient data to assess the value of psychotherapy in persons with ASPD.

The correct response is option E: There are insufficient data to assess the value of psychotherapy in persons with ASPD.

According to the National Institute for Health and Clinical Excellence and the Cochrane Database reviews, the data are insufficient to assess the value of psychotherapy in persons with ASPD (Gibbon et al. 2010). Complicating these reviews is the fact that most studies reviewed involved participants other than those with ASPD. **(p. 446)**

References

Black DW: Bad Boys, Bad Men: Confronting Antisocial Personality Disorder (Sociopathy), Revised and Updated. New York, Oxford University Press, 2013

Black DW, Baumgard CH, Bell SE: A 16- to 45-year follow-up of 71 men with antisocial personality disorder. Compr Psychiatry 36:130–140, 1995a 7758299

Black DW, Baumgard CH, Bell SE: The long-term outcome of antisocial personality disorder compared with depression, schizophrenia, and surgical conditions. Bull Am Acad Psychiatry Law 23:43–52, 1995b 7599370

Brennan PA, Mednick SA: Genetic perspectives on crime. Acta Psychiatr Scand Suppl 370:19–26, 1993 8452051

Burt SA, Donnellan MB, Humbad MN, et al: Does marriage inhibit antisocial behavior? An examination of selection vs causation via a longitudinal twin design. Arch Gen Psychiatry 67:1309–1315, 2010 21135331

Cadoret RJ, O'Gorman TW, Troughton E, et al: Alcoholism and antisocial personality: interrelationships, genetic and environmental factors. Arch Gen Psychiatry 42:161–167, 1985 3977542

Caspi A, McClay J, Moffitt TE, et al: Role of genotype in the cycle of violence in maltreated children. Science 297:851–854, 2002 12161658

Compton WM, Conway KP, Stinson FS, et al: Prevalence, correlates, and comorbidity of DSM-IV antisocial personality syndromes and alcohol and specific drug use disorders in the United States: results from the National Epidemiologic Survey on Alcohol and Related Conditions. J Clin Psychiatry 66:677–685, 2005 15960559

Gibbon S, Duggan C, Stoffers J, et al: Psychological interventions for antisocial personality disorder. Cochrane Database of Systematic Reviews 2010, Issue 6. Art. No.: CD007668. DOI: 10. 1002/14651858.CD007668.pub2.

Goldstein RB, Dawson DA, Saha TD, et al: Antisocial behavioral syndromes and DSM-IV alcohol use disorders: results from the National Epidemiologic Survey on Alcohol and Related Conditions. Alcohol Clin Exp Res 31:814–828, 2007 17391341

Guze SB, Wolfgram ED, McKinney JK, et al: Psychiatric illness in the families of convicted criminals: a study of 519 first-degree relatives. Dis Nerv Syst 28:651–659, 1967 6051292

Hare RD: Twenty years of experience with the Cleckley psychopath, in Unmasking the Psychopath—Antisocial Personality and Related Syndromes. Edited by Reid WJ, Dorr D, Walker JI, et al. New York, WW Norton, 1986, pp 3–27

National Collaborating Centre for Mental Health: Antisocial Personality Disorder: Treatment, Management, and Prevention. The National Institute for Health and Clinical Excellence (NICE) Guidelines. National Clinical Practice Guideline No 77. London, RCPsych Publications, 2009

Raine A, Lencz T, Bihrle S, et al: Reduced prefrontal gray matter volume and reduced autonomic activity and antisocial personality disorder. Arch Gen Psychiatry 57:119–127, 2000 10665614

Robins LN: Deviant Children Grown Up: A Sociological and Psychiatric Study of Sociopathic Personality. Baltimore, MD, Williams & Wilkins, 1966

Robins LN: The epidemiology of antisocial personality disorder, in Psychiatry, Vol 3. Edited by Michels RO, Cavenar JO. Philadelphia, PA, Lippincott, 1987, pp 1–14

Robins LN, Price RK: Adult disorders predicted by childhood conduct problems: results from the NIMH Epidemiologic Catchment Area project. Psychiatry 54:116–132, 1991 1852846

Sampson R, Laub J: Crime in the Making: Pathways and Turning Points Through Life. Cambridge, MA, Harvard University Press, 1993

Scarpa A, Raine A: Psychophysiology of anger and violent behavior. Psychiatr Clin North Am 20:375–403, 1997 9196920

Slutske WS: The genetics of antisocial behavior. Curr Psychiatry Rep 3:158–162, 2001 11276412

Ullrich S, Coid J: Antisocial personality disorder: co-morbid Axis I mental disorders and health service use among a national household population. Personality and Mental Health 3:151–164, 2009

Yang Y, Raine A, Narr KL, et al: Localisation of prefrontal white matter in pathological liars. Br J Psychiatry 190:174–175, 2007 17267937

Yang Y, Raine A, Narr KL, et al: Localization of deformations within the amygdala of individuals with psychopathy. Arch Gen Psychiatry 66:986–994, 2009 19736355

CHAPTER 21

Personality Disorders in the Medical Setting

21.1   Which of the following is particularly indicative of personality dysfunction in a medical outpatient?

A. A patient who is experienced as "difficult."
B. Disruptive behaviors that have persisted over many years.
C. Unacceptable behavior by a patient recently given a distressing diagnosis.
D. Clinic staff liking the patient very much.
E. A patient who carefully researches the medical diagnosis.

The correct response is option B: Disruptive behaviors that have persisted over many years.

Patients in medical settings may display a number of behaviors that are *suggestive* of personality pathology. When these behaviors are clinically present, the clinician should consider an assessment for personality pathology. The longitudinal nature or pervasiveness of behaviors is particularly indicative of the presence of personality dysfunction. The presence of repetitive or long-standing patterns of disruptive behaviors supports the diagnosis of personality pathology, whereas novel fleeting behaviors are caused by contemporary psychosocial stressors, medications, and/or the illness itself and would not suggest a personality disorder (PD) (option C). "Difficult" patients (option A) may be patients with PDs, but many patients may be characterized as difficult, including patients with somatic symptom disorders, mood disorders, and psychoses. Patients with PDs are often disliked by the clinic staff (option D), and a patient who researches his or her diagnosis without being disruptive to the medical care does not indicate a personality diagnosis (option E). **(p. 457)**

21.2   Research on patients with borderline PD (BPD) in the medical setting indicates that which of the following are common behaviors?

A. Seductive approaches to the clinic staff.
B. Life-threatening remarks to the clinic staff.
C. Unusual openness and willingness to talk with the clinic staff.

D. Yelling and screaming at the clinic staff.

E. Frequent compliments about the clinic to family.

The correct response is option D: Yelling and screaming at the clinic staff.

In an effort to clarify the range of poor patient conduct in medical settings, Sansone et al. (2011) explored in a survey of internal medicine outpatients the prevalence of 17 disruptive behaviors as well as their relationship to borderline personality symptomatology. They found that the number of different types of disruptive office behaviors reported by participants was statistically significantly correlated with both self-report measures for BPD used in this study. Compared with participants without borderline personality symptomatology, patients with such symptoms were significantly more likely to report yelling, screaming, verbal threats, and/or refusing to talk to medical personnel (options A, C) as well as talking disrespectfully about medical personnel to both family and friends (option E) (Sansone et al. 2011). Note that although the preceding behaviors are clearly intimidating and demoralizing for treatment providers as well as disruptive to the patient/clinician environment, they are not necessarily life-threatening to the clinician (option B). **(pp. 458–459)**

21.3   Which PD is most closely correlated with intentional sabotage of medical care?

A. Paranoid PD.

B. Dependent PD.

C. Avoidant PD.

D. BPD.

E. Schizotypal PD.

The correct response is option D: BPD.

Intentionally sabotaging one's own medical care is a phenomenon that has been recognized for some time, through clinical experience as well as occasional case reports and small empirical studies (e.g., factitious disorder). However, links between medical sabotage and specific types of personality pathology have only recently been clarified. A prime PD contender for the intentional sabotage of one's own medical care is BPD, because this type of behavior may function as a self-injury equivalent (Sansone and Sansone 2012b). However, antisocial PD cannot be excluded, particularly if the intent of medical sabotage serves some illicit purpose such as the procurement of narcotic analgesics with the intent to sell them.

One syndrome related to factitious disorder is intentionally making medical situations worse. Sansone and Wiederman (2009a) have confirmed the relationships between intentionally making medical situations worse and borderline personality symptomatology. Explicitly, they examined a compiled sample of databases and scrutinized the subsample that consisted of internal medicine outpatient only ($n=332$). In this subsample, 16.7% of participants acknowledged intentionally making medical situations worse, and this phenomenon demonstrated a statistically significant relationship with the measure for borderline personality symptomatology that was used in the study. **(p. 459)**

21.4 An obstetrical colleague stops you in the hallway to ask about a patient she recently admitted for a nonhealing wound following an emergency caesarean section several weeks ago. She asks, "Could she be intentionally trying to not let the wound heal?" The patient uses only acetaminophen for pain but is demanding that the nursing staff get her special foods. What is the most likely PD diagnosis for this patient?

A. Antisocial.
B. Paranoid.
C. Narcissistic.
D. Borderline.
E. Dependent.

The correct response is option D: Borderline.

Preventing wounds from healing—another form of medical self-sabotage——has been empirically investigated in relationship to personality dysfunction. At the outset, the idea of preventing wounds from healing is somewhat disconcerting, but the phenomenon is not particularly rare in clinical populations. For example, Sansone and Sansone (2012b) found modest prevalence rates in various types of clinical samples (i.e., between 0.8% in cardiac-stress-test patients and 4.2% in internal medicine outpatients). With regard to links to personality pathology, in a consecutive sample of internal medicine outpatients, an obstetrics/gynecology sample, and a sample of four compiled databases, they consistently found statistically significant relationships between intentionally preventing wounds from healing and borderline personality symptomatology (Sansone and Wiederman 2009b; Sansone et al. 2010, 2012). This association may be the manifestation of a typical borderline patient's intense needs to be taken care of. **(pp. 459–460)**

21.5 In what situation would the "Headlines Test" be useful for a primary care physician taking care of a patient?

A. When referring the patient for a psychiatric consultation.
B. When confronting the patient about provocative dress.
C. When telling the patient to stop offering free tickets to the clinic staff.
D. When using the state's online program to check if the patient is obtaining controlled substances from several different physicians.
E. When accepting the patient's invitation to see the Kentucky Derby in the family's private box.

The correct response is option E: When accepting the patient's invitation to see the Kentucky Derby in the family's private box.

When the clinician is unsure about how to respond to a patient's provocative behavior, he or she should consider the "Headlines Test"—that is, how the clinician's behavior would appear to the public if it were publicized in the headlines of the local newspaper. With time and experience in the clinical setting, clinicians gradually discern the range of appropriate behaviors that are acceptable in the clinician-patient relationship. As expected, this range of sanctioned behaviors corresponds to an associated set of interpersonal boundaries as well. Unfortunately, individuals with PDs (e.g., narcissistic PD and/or BPD) often have intense needs to disrupt these professional boundaries—perhaps to be uniquely "known" by the clinician, to be perceived as "the special patient" in the medical setting, and/or to be "loved." These intense needs by the patient can, at times, manifest as overtly inappropriate behaviors and may include sexual innuendos, provocative clothing and/or body displays, awkward solicitations for social outings, inappropriate or premature address of the clinician by first name, excessive or expensive gift giving, and/or requests for special services or "favors." Clinicians need to be extremely wary of inappropriately resonating with these types of boundary violations, because to do so may lead to further deterioration in the boundaries of the professional relationship (i.e., an escalating need by the patient for repeated affirmations). These boundary disturbances may ultimately culminate in clinician entrapment and/or legal consequences. Option E is clearly a situation that does not pass the Headlines Test. Options A, B, C, and D deal with limit setting or are appropriate even if published in the newspaper. **(p. 460)**

21.6 Which of the following statements correctly describes the relationship between chronic pain and PDs?

A. Younger patients with BPD are more likely to report chronic pain than older patients with BPD.
B. Patients with BPD rarely report chronic pain syndromes.
C. Medical disability is considerably higher in chronic pain patients with BPD compared with those without PD.
D. Medical disability is considerably lower in chronic pain patients with BPD compared with those without PD.
E. Medical disability is no different in chronic pain patients with BPD compared with those without PD.

The correct response is option E: Medical disability is no different in chronic pain patients with BPD compared with those without PD.

Chronic pain is a globally complex issue, including its relationship with personality dysfunction. In the context of PDs, chronic pain may be the psychodynamic outgrowth of magnification, helplessness, and/or rumination (i.e., alterations in the actual perception and/or experience of pain); the inability to effectively self-regulate pain; a covert attempt to elicit caring responses from health care professionals; a means of maintaining a disabled status (i.e., a self-defeating lifestyle); and/or a means of procuring prescription medications for illicit purposes. Because of these varying factors, chronic pain syndromes may encompass a number of different types of individuals with personality dysfunction, especially borderline and antisocial PDs. In a literature review, Sansone and Sansone (2012a) examined the prevalence of BPD among samples of individuals with various types of chronic pain syndromes. They encountered eight studies since 1994 and found that the average prevalence rate for BPD among these samples was 30% (option B). Individuals with BPD reported higher levels of pain than participants without BPD; older individuals with BPD, rather than younger individuals, were more likely to report higher pain levels (option A); and the first-degree relatives of participants with BPD demonstrated statistical coaggregation with somatoform pain disorder. Unexpectedly, they also found that the prevalence of medical disability did *not* differ substantially among chronic-pain participants with versus without BPD (options C, D). **(p. 463)**

21.7   What is the goal for the psychiatric consultant for a patient with a PD who is disruptive and uncooperative during an acute medical admission?

A. Engage the patient in psychotherapy to treat the PD.
B. Focus on the unit staff having problematic interactions with the patient to elucidate what is realistically problematic about his or her behavior.
C. Avoid the use of psychotropic medication at all costs.
D. Stabilize the patient in order to complete the medical evaluation and necessary treatment.
E. Take as long as it is necessary to assess the situation and arrive at a plan.

The correct response is option D: Stabilize the patient in order to complete the medical evaluation and necessary treatment.

With regard to intervention, the clinical situation may at times be promptly resolved by clarifying limits (i.e., "We need to complete this test by the end of the day"), particularly if family support is available (Dhossche and Shevitz 1999). Brief negotiation and/or verbal contracting with the patient may be helpful (Pare and Rosenbluth 1999). The acute use of psychotropic medications (e.g., antipsychotics) with rapid-onset effects may be indicated to either calm and/or reorganize the patient (option C). It may also be crucial to clear up any distortions in communication between the patient and staff (Norton 2000). In addition, if the patient is directing detrimental commentary to specific staff members, these individuals need to be informed to deflect the negative content on a personal level, despite the very personal intent by the patient (option B) (Pare and Rosenbluth 1999). Finally, the consulting clinician may need to reinforce boundaries between the patient and staff (Devens 2007), which may entail the reassignment of the patient to another provider or nursing staff member or even transferring the patient to another medical service or to a mental health facility. The key strategy during the acute consultation is to quickly assess the situation and review and suggest available options for intervention (option E). In acute patient-care situations, immediate and reasonable stabilization of the patient is mandated in order to complete the medical task. The goal is not the treatment of the patient's personality pathology (option A). Ideally, the clinician is hoping to pacify the patient so that the clinical situation will conclude successfully (i.e., the clinician and treatment team will be able to provide the appropriate and indicated medical assessment and care). **(p. 467)**

21.8   Which of the following personal physician characteristics may cause unintentional problems in treating patients with PDs in the longitudinal patient-care situation?

A. A physician who is psychosocially minded.
B. Personal physician characteristics have no impact on the relationship with patients who have PDs.
C. A physician who has a clear concept of his or her personal responsibility in the clinical outcome.
D. A physician who shows no response to a patient's intense emotions and passively withdraws from the patient.
E. A physician who feels comfortable with what is and what is not appropriate patient behavior.

The correct response is option D: A physician who shows no response to a patient's intense emotions and passively withdraws from the patient.

On occasion, the clinician's personal qualities and attitudes may be unintentionally contributing to the difficulties in his or her relationship with the patient. Although less relevant in the acute patient-care situation, the clinician-patient relationship is paramount in the longitudinal patient-care situation (option B). In this regard, Meyer and Block (2011) broach a number of important points. They indicate that less psychosocially minded clinicians are more prone to reporting difficult encounters with patients (option A). In addition, patients with more severe PDs tend to evoke stronger emotions in clinicians, and these emotions may be expressed by the clinician in problematic ways toward the patient. For example, clinicians who underrespond to the intense emotions of patients by passively withdrawing may cause undue patient distress related to feelings of abandonment. Alternatively, clinicians who actively respond to the strong emotions of patients with brusqueness or confrontation may unintentionally distance the patient. In addition, Meyer and Block (2011) emphasize that some clinicians may struggle with their own personal concepts of appropriate and inappropriate behaviors during patient encounters (option E), be vexed by their sense of personal responsibility for a positive outcome in a seemingly uncooperative patient (option C), and/ or be overly attached to the concept of "tireless caregiver" and wind up feeling emotionally exhausted by a demanding patient. The key consideration for the consultant is to entertain the clinician's possible role in a patient-management issue, which may not only acutely alleviate the current situation but also prevent future crises. **(p. 468)**

21.9   What is the role of the clinician's experience in medicine in dealing effectively with patients who have PDs?

A. Early-career physicians deal more effectively with these patients than do experienced physicians.
B. The idealization of the practice of medicine common early in a physician's career aids in effective management of patients with PDs.
C. The clinical impasses that occur with these patients do not bother early-career physicians.
D. More experienced physicians are less susceptible to unrealistic expectations of themselves and are better able to handle the difficulties involved in treating patients with PDs.
E. Experience does not influence how physicians handle the difficulties involved in treating patients with PDs.

The correct response is option D: More experienced physicians are less susceptible to unrealistic expectations of themselves and are better able to handle the difficulties involved in treating patients with PDs.

Pare and Rosenbluth (1999) discuss the role of the clinician's experience in medicine and the resulting impact on his or her expectations of medical practice in relationships with patients. At the outset, newly trained clinicians tend to initially idealize the practice of medicine. Many are initially attracted to the field of medicine because they are driven by their own deep needs to help others and to feel effective and potent while doing so. Unfortunately, patients with dramatic personality dysfunction tend to leave clinicians feeling ineffective and impotent (options A, B, C), particularly when derailing the treatment course with noncompliance, eruptions of disruptive behavior, and demands for unnecessary and potentially harmful medications. These types of clinical impasses with patients tend to compromise the obsessive-compulsive mindset of many young clinicians by thwarting their efforts to "do the right thing" for the patient. With time in the field, a more realistic perspective begins to gradually evolve (option E). Pare and Rosenbluth (1999) stress that "all" clinicians eventually learn that "medicine is not as powerful and effective as they had hoped it would be" (p. 262), suggesting that with seasoning, clinicians will be less susceptible to these kinds of initial unrealistic expectations of the practice of medicine. **(pp. 468–469)**

21.10 An internal medicine colleague asks to talk to you about a patient she has followed for 5 years. She recognized at the beginning of treatment that her patient had BPD from the patient's history of chaotic relationships, cutting behaviors, substance abuse, and impulsivity; however, she felt she could manage the patient because her medical condition was one in which the physician was an expert. She has seen the patient biweekly, usually for short visits. Over the past 6 months, she has seen the patient weekly for 30- to 60-minute visits, during which they discuss the patient's relationships. She feels she approaches the patient calmly, even when the patient is unreasonable and monitors for when the patient is seeking extra analgesics or discusses pursuing therapies that might be harmful medically. When the patient has been disruptive in the clinic, the physician has worked with her and the staff to resolve the issues, even though the staff has wanted the patient to be discharged from the clinic. During the 5 years of treatment, the patient complained about the internist's vacations, but last month while the internist was away, the patient cut herself and required stitches to repair the wound. In reviewing the case, what is the mistake that the internist is making in the management of this patient?

A. Attempting to do psychotherapy with the patient.
B. Not discharging the patient from the clinic.
C. Discussing the patient's seeking potentially harmful medical treatments.
D. Involving multiple physicians in the patient's care.
E. Seeing the patient biweekly for many years.

The correct response is option A: Attempting to do psychotherapy with the patient.

The recommended overall management approach to patients with PDs in the medical setting entails a broad menu of options. Suggested options for the clinician include 1) maintaining an emotionally neutral treatment environment (e.g., self-monitoring one's responses to the patient, avoiding the direct expression of anger, not making personal comments); 2) being supportive to the patient; 3) limiting in-office attempts at psychotherapy; 4) scheduling multiple brief appointments to address the needs of those individuals who struggle with strong attachment dynamics (option E); and 5) preventing the patient from getting into high-risk medical situations, that is, maintaining conservative medical management (option C). These high-risk medical situations may include the unnecessary prescription of scheduled and potentially harmful medications (e.g., narcotic analgesics, controlled weight-loss medications, stimulants for attention-deficit/hyperactivity disorder, controlled anxiolytic medications), unnecessary laboratory studies (i.e., given a sufficient number of laboratory studies, occasional spurious results are bound to occur, creating more challenges in the treatment), and unnecessary referrals to specialists (option D) for invasive diagnostic procedures or treatments (i.e., some specialists may not be aware of the nature of personality pathology and may unintentionally overtreat patients with PDs). In addition, the centering of care in the medical office enables the streamlining of patient management by maintaining clearly defined treatment goals, including a clear explanation of the treatment plan to the patient, and a consistent treatment provider ("one cook in the kitchen"). Because of this, patient visits to the emergency room are to be discouraged except in a genuine emergency. Establishing a treatment milieu in which symptom resolution is deemed unlikely is encouraged, but symptom management is the more realistic treatment goal (e.g., "We are never going to rid you of your pain, but we can reduce the amount of pain") (Dhossche and Shevitz 1999).

Although it may seem appealing to discharge difficult patients from one's medical practice, it may actually be in the patient's best interest to remain in the practice, particularly if the interpersonal situation between the clinician and patient can be stabilized (option B). On occasion, patients with PDs may seek atypical treatments from unprofessional treatment resources—a situation that should be avoided at the outset to protect the patient. **(pp. 469–470)**

References

Devens M: Personality disorders. Prim Care 34:623–640, 2007 17868763

Dhossche DM, Shevitz SA: Assessment and importance of personality disorders in medical patients: an update. South Med J 92:546–556, 1999 10372846

Meyer F, Block S: Personality disorders in the oncology setting. J Support Oncol 9:44–51, 2011 21542408

Norton JW: Personality disorders in the primary care setting. Nurse Pract 25:40–42, 51, 55–58, 2000 11149142

Pare MF, Rosenbluth M: Personality disorders in primary care. Prim Care 26:243–278, 1999 10318747

Sansone RA, Sansone LA: Chronic pain syndromes and borderline personality. Innov Clin Neurosci 9:10–14, 2012a 22347686

Sansone RA, Sansone LA: Medically self-sabotaging behavior and its relationship with borderline personality. Prim Care Rep 18:37–47, 2012b

Sansone RA, Wiederman MW: Making medical situations worse: patient disclosures in psychiatric versus medical settings. J Med 2:169–171, 2009a

Sansone RA, Wiederman MW: Interference with wound healing: borderline patients in psychiatric versus medical settings. Prim Care Companion J Clin Psychiatry 11:271–272, 2009b 19956470

Sansone RA, Lam C, Wiederman MW: The abuse of prescription medications: a relationship with borderline personality? J Opioid Manag 6:159–160, 2010 20642243

Sansone RA, Farukhi S, Wiederman MW: Disruptive behaviors in the medical setting and borderline personality. Int J Psychiatry Med 41:355–363, 2011 22238840

Sansone RA, Lam C, Wiederman MW: Hairpulling and borderline personality symptomatology among internal medicine outpatients. Intern Med J 42:345–347, 2012 22432993

CHAPTER 22

Personality Disorders in the Military Operational Environment

22.1   Which of the following statements about military service is true?

    A. Military leaders are not required to attempt to correct deficiencies and rehabilitate behavior that is detrimental to occupational and social functioning within the military.

    B. Establishment of a diagnosis of a personality disorder (PD) after enlistment is viewed as a condition that did not exist prior to enlistment.

    C. Behavioral health care is not available to military personnel with PDs.

    D. The military does not allow for relatively expeditious administrative separation of service members with PDs.

    E. Stressors in military life may precipitate episodes of decompensation in service members with PDs.

The correct response is option E: Stressors in military life may precipitate episodes of decompensation in service members with PDs.

The U.S. military has long recognized that persons with behavioral or interpersonal impairments that are commonly manifested in PDs may be poorly suited for military duty. Both military culture and military regulations require that leaders must strive to correct the deficiencies in their service members and to rehabilitate behavior that is detrimental to occupational or social functioning within the military (e.g., through mentoring, corrective training, or even nonjudicial punishment) (option A). Behavioral health care, ranging from medication management to individual and group supportive, psychoeducational, cognitive-behavioral, and in some cases intensive psychodynamic psychotherapy, is available to service members who seek treatment for mental disorders within a wide variety of treatment facilities on military bases and during deployment (option C). However, in recognition of the traditional view of the ingrained and enduring nature of PD related behaviors and the barriers to effective treatment of PDs imposed by occupational requirements of military service (e.g., ready access to weapons, frequent moves, short-notice deployment to locations without the full panoply of psychiatric resources), all branches of the military also promulgate regulations that allow for relatively expeditious administrative separation (without disability compensation) of service members with PDs (option D). The diagnosis of PD serves as a bar to enlistment, and the emergence of a PD diagnosis after enlistment is viewed, from a disability compensation standpoint, as the recognition of a condition that existed prior to enlistment (option B). More recent studies suggest that personality disordered behavior is more waxing and waning than it is enduring; the recurrent nature of the stressors inherent to military life may precipitate episodes of decompensation rather than protect against them. **(pp. 476–477)**

22.2   Which of the following statements concerning medical and psychological screening for enlistment to military service is true?

   A. The U.S. military conducts formal, comprehensive psychiatric and psychological screening tests on all persons entering active military service.
   B. PD diagnoses documented prior to entry into the military serve as bars to enlistment.
   C. Specialized military occupations (e.g., Special Forces) are prohibited from using formal psychological screening for enlistment and selection.
   D. Complete psychological/psychiatric histories are always obtained during the enlistment process.
   E. Prevalence rates for military personnel with PDs are well established and can be used to guide enlistment.

   The correct response is option B: PD diagnoses documented prior to entry into the military serve as bars to enlistment.

   The U.S. military does not conduct comprehensive psychiatric or psychological screening on all persons entering active duty or such surveillance on any periodic basis after entry into active duty (option A). Some specialized military occupations (e.g., Special Forces or recruiting duties) may use psychological screening for assessment and selection purposes, but these represent exceptions rather than the norm for military duty (option C). Military accession standards preclude persons with a variety of medical illnesses, including chronic psychotic disorders, substance use disorders, and PDs, from enlistment, and documented histories of these illnesses serve as bars to initial enlistment. However, if such histories are not reported on enlistment applications or in medical records reviewed prior to enlistment, they may be missed (option D). Therefore, prevalence rates for psychiatric diagnoses that do not necessarily come to clinical attention (including PDs) have not been clearly established (option E). **(p. 477)**

22.3   Which of the following is NOT a standard pathway to mental health care for active duty service members with personality disorders?

   A. Service members may obtain a primary care referral to see a mental health specialist.

B. Service members with PDs may self-refer for behavioral health care.

C. Commanders or supervisors may encourage service members to seek mental health treatment.

D. Peers may refer or accompany fellow service members to behavioral health care.

E. All service members receive behavioral health care as a standard component of their medical care.

The correct response is option E: All service members receive behavioral health care as a standard component of their medical care.

Service members with PDs may present to either primary care physicians or mental health specialists (option A) for assistance in times of emotional crisis (e.g., suicidal ideation when a deployment threatens the security of a romantic relationship, excessive anger or depressed mood after failing to receive a promotion). In other circumstances, maladaptive behaviors (e.g., impulsive aggression, substance misuse, disregard for direct orders, self-injurious acts) may be directly observed by or reported to commanders by subordinates concerned for the safety of the service member. Others in the command may become concerned that a mental disorder may be jeopardizing a service member's ability to carry out his or her mission. Commanders, supervisors, or peers may certainly encourage fellow service members to seek mental health treatment in these circumstances (options C, D). Considerable effort has been invested by the services in promoting the concept that service members should actively encourage their colleagues to seek treatment or counseling voluntarily when such concerns arise. Behavioral health care is available to any service member who requests it (option B), although it is not provided routinely. **(pp. 479–480)**

22.4   Systematic health surveillance studies conducted by the Mental Health Advisory Team (MHAT) during combat operations in Iraq and Afghanistan demonstrated a significant increase in the prevalence of which of the following diagnoses during and after deployment when compared with garrison or predeployment rates?

A. Major depression, substance use disorders, and posttraumatic stress disorder (PTSD).

B. PTSD, substance use disorders, and psychotic disorders.

C. PDs, PTSD, and substance use disorders.

D. Major depression, substance use disorders, and psychotic disorders.

E. Substance use disorders, PDs, and major depression.

The correct response is option A: Major depression, substance use disorders, and posttraumatic stress disorder (PTSD).

Systematic health surveillance efforts in Iraq and Afghanistan such as those conducted by the MHAT have compiled considerable data on the prevalence of psychiatric disorders in combat personnel. The MHAT studies rely heavily on anonymous self-report questionnaires through which service members report symptoms experienced at the time of survey administration. These studies have demonstrated significant increases in rates of diagnoses including major depression, PTSD, and substance use disorders at 3 months, 6 months, and 1 year following deployment, as well as increased prevalence of these disorders during deployment when compared with garrison or predeployment rates (Hoge et al. 2004). **(pp. 477–478)**

22.5 Systematic examination of military health care utilization revealed that incidence rates of which diagnoses remained generally stable or declined between the years 2000 and 2011?

  A. Substance use disorders and adjustment disorders.
  B. Psychotic disorders and PDs.
  C. Adjustment disorders and PTSD.
  D. PDs and anxiety disorders.
  E. Major depression and adjustment disorders.

The correct response is option B: Psychotic disorders and PDs.

One recently published systematic examination of military health utilization databases showed that from 2000 to 2011, a total of 936,283 service members received at least one mental disorder diagnosis at a military treatment facility, and nearly half had more than one (Armed Forces Health Surveillance Center 2012). Not surprisingly, incidence rates of PTSD, anxiety disorders, depressive disorders, adjustment disorders, and other mental disorders generally increased during this time period (with adjustment disorders accounting for 85% of all incident diagnoses and incidence rates of PTSD increasing approximately sixfold). However, over the entire period, relatively few incident diagnoses were attributable to PDs ($n=81,223$). The incidence rate for the diagnostic category PD—which comprised all subtypes, including mixed—was generally stable at approximately 500 cases/100,000 person-years and actually declined slightly over the period of study ($n=8,281$ in 2001; $n=4,110$ in 2011). Similarly stable patterns were observed for psychotic disorders and substance abuse and dependence disorders. See Figure 22–1 provided here. **(pp. 478–479)**

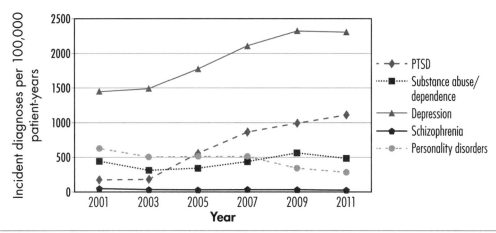

Incidence rates of mental disorder diagnoses, by category, active component, U.S. Armed Forces, 2001–2011.

Source. Adapted from "Mental Disorders and Mental Health Problems, Active Component, U.S. Armed Forces, 2000–2011." *Medical Surveillance Monthly Report* 19(6):13, 2012.

22.6 Conditions that render a service member *unsuitable* for military service differ from conditions that render a service member *unfit* for military service in which of the following ways?

    A. The terms *unsuitable* and *unfit* are interchangeable designations that do not affect benefits after separation from the military.

    B. Determining a service member *unsuitable* for military service allows for medical retirement with benefits.

    C. Determining a service member *unfit* for military service may result in administrative separation without benefits.

    D. Conditions that can render a service member *unsuitable* for military service include PDs, enuresis, motion sickness, and sleepwalking.

    E. Conditions that can render a service member *unfit* for military service include PDs, enuresis, motion sickness, and sleepwalking.

The correct response is option D: Conditions that can render a service member *unsuitable* for military service include PDs, enuresis, motion sickness, and sleepwalking.

Historically, service regulations have addressed conditions that are considered *unsuitable* for military service but that do not necessarily render the service member *unfit* for military service (i.e., not amounting to disability) (options A, B). These include such conditions as enuresis and motion sickness, as well as behavioral conditions that would limit the person's ability to adapt to the demands of military service but not otherwise interfere with routine civilian life activities. This regulation allowed for the administrative separation of soldiers demonstrating "a deeply ingrained maladaptive pattern of behavior that interferes with the

Soldier's ability to perform duty" (U.S. Department of the Army 2011, p. 58). Service regulations that address conditions considered unsuitable for military service (U.S. Department of the Air Force 2011; U.S. Department of the Army 2011; U.S. Department of the Navy 2009) are derived from U.S. Department of Defense (2011) policy. As previously noted, these include conditions such as motion sickness, enuresis, and sleepwalking, which would not generally be considered disabling but which could obviously be incompatible with military service (option E). In the case of physical illness, injury, or major mental disorders incurred or exacerbated while on active duty or service, the conditions leading to medical retirement (to include disability compensation) are articulated in the regulations of the U. S. Department of the Army, the instructions of the U.S. Department of the Air Force, and in the manual of the U.S. Navy's Medical Department. The procedures for disability processing, only after a member has received maximum degree of medical benefit from acute treatment, are enumerated in "Physical Disability Evaluation" (U.S. Department of Defense Instruction 2006). Medical retirement indicates a service member is unfit for active duty (option C). **(pp. 481–482)**

22.7   Who makes the final disposition about a service member's administrative separation from service?

A. A military psychiatrist.
B. A military court-martial.
C. The service member's commander.
D. A Medical Evaluation Board.
E. The service member.

The correct response is option C: The service member's commander.

The regulations provide that even with the diagnosis of a PD, a recommendation for administrative separation remains only a recommendation, with final disposition determined by the commander only after "the Soldier has been counseled formally concerning deficiencies and has been afforded ample opportunity to overcome those deficiencies as reflected in appropriate counseling or personnel records" (U.S. Department of the Army 2011, p. 56). This guidance is in keeping with the special emphasis the military places on mentorship and leadership and is consistent with military values exhorting leaders to exhaust efforts to rehabilitate deficiencies in their subordinates before giving up on them. **(p. 482)**

22.8   Recommendations from the Army Task Force on Behavioral Health led to which changes in disability evaluations in military service members in 2011?

A. They allowed disability evaluations to consider behavioral changes that might stem from PDs or adjustment disorders to be eligible solely for administrative separation instead of medical disability compensation.
B. They allowed disability evaluations to consider behavioral changes that may stem from trauma and combat to be eligible solely for administrative separation instead of medical disability compensation.

C. They designated specific guidelines about the conducting of psychological evaluations.
D. They discontinued all administrative separations for behavioral changes in active duty members.
E. They allowed disability evaluations to consider behavioral changes that might stem from PDs and adjustment disorders to be considered in a light that would be most beneficial to the service member in terms of potential disability compensation instead of administrative separation.

The correct response is option E: They allowed disability evaluations to consider behavioral changes that might stem from PDs and adjustment disorders to be considered in a light that would be most beneficial to the service member in terms of potential disability compensation instead of administrative separation.

In late 2011, concerns were raised about Medical Evaluation Board evaluations of psychiatric conditions conducted at Madigan Army Medical Center at Joint Base Lewis-McChord in Washington State. This eventually resulted in the establishment of the Army Task Force on Behavioral Health, chartered to conduct a comprehensive evaluation of the Disability Evaluation System in an effort to "review, assess, and, where needed, improve behavioral health evaluations in the context of Disability Evaluation System" (Army Task Force on Behavioral Health 2013, p. 7). The task force made a number of recommendations regarding processes to improve the efficiency of the disability evaluation system, as well as indicated the need to educate service members and clinicians regarding the diagnostic assessment process. The goals of the recommended changes are to enhance the comprehensiveness of the assessment process and to ensure careful evaluation of all symptoms, including behavioral changes that might stem from PD or adjustment disorder. Although specific guidelines about the conduct of evaluations were not made (options C), the process allows these behavioral changes to be considered in a light that would be most beneficial to the service member in terms of potential disability compensation versus administrative separation (options A, B, D). **(p. 483)**

22.9 Which of the following diagnostic categories has sufficient overlap of symptoms with PD symptoms, potentially leading to the misdiagnosis and administrative separation of military service members?

A. Traumatic brain injury.
B. Schizophrenia.
C. Sleep-wake cycle disorders.
D. Bereavement.
E. Major depression.

The correct response is option A: Traumatic brain injury.

There has been increasing awareness that frequent and prolonged deployment with associated disruption of social support, repeated exposure to harsh environments and life-threatening situations, and physical trauma stresses all service members, including those with identifiable PDs. The military has invested considerable effort in the development of better approaches to the assessment and management of PTSD, traumatic brain injury, and the interpersonal and occupational impairments that may result from these disorders. These efforts have also resulted in an increased awareness of the diagnostic overlap not only between these entities but also with adjustment disorders and PDs, as each of these may manifest in patterns of maladaptive behavior that may only come to clinical attention with the added stressors of deployment and redeployment. **(p. 484)**

References

Armed Forces Health Surveillance Center: Mental disorders and mental health problems, active component, U.S. Armed Forces, 2000–2011. Medical Surveillance Monthly Report 19(6):11–17, 2012. Available at: http://www.afhsc.mil/viewMSMR?file=2012/v19_n06.pdf. Accessed March 15, 2014.

Army Task Force on Behavioral Health: Corrective Action Plan, January 2013. Available at: http://s3.documentcloud.org/documents/613090/atfbh-corrective-action-plan-5-march-13.pdf. Accessed March 15, 2014.

Bollinger AR, Riggs DS, Blake DD, et al: Prevalence of personality disorders among combat veterans with posttraumatic stress disorder. J Trauma Stress 13:255–270, 2000 10838674

Hoge CW, Castro CA, Messer SC, et al: Combat duty in Iraq and Afghanistan, mental health problems, and barriers to care. N Engl J Med 351:3–22, 2004 15229303

U.S. Department of Defense Instruction: Physical disability evaluation (1332.38), 2006. Available at: http://www.dtic.mil/whs/directives/corres/pdf/133238p.pdf. Accessed August 27, 2013

U.S. Department of the Air Force: Administrative Separation of Airmen (Air Force Instruction [AFI] 36-3208). Washington, DC, Department of the Air Force, 2011

U.S. Department of the Army: Active Duty Enlisted Administrative Separations (Army Regulation 635-200). Washington, DC, Department of the Army, 2011

U.S. Department of Defense Instruction: Enlisted administrative separations (1332.14), 2011. Available at: http://www.dtic.mil/whs/directives/corres/pdf/133214p.pdf. Accessed March 15, 2014.

U.S. Department of the Navy: U.S. Navy MILPERSMAN: Separation by reason of convenience of the government—personality disorder(s) (1910-122), August 2009. Available at: http://www.public.navy.mil/bupers-npc/reference/milpersman/1000/1900Separation/Documents/1910-122.pdf. Accessed March 15, 2014.

CHAPTER 23

Translational Research in Borderline Personality Disorder

23.1   Which of the following phenotypes of borderline personality disorder (BPD) described by Gunderson and colleagues is its most distinctive and pathogenic component?

   A. Antisocial traits.
   B. Self-loathing.
   C. Interpersonal hypersensitivity.
   D. Rejection projection.
   E. Provider idealization.

The correct response is option C: Interpersonal hypersensitivity.

Gunderson et al. (2007) emphasized "the fearful or highly reactive component of this interpersonal style that is probably the more distinctive and pathogenic component" (p. 2) of BPD and referred to this interpersonal style as the interpersonal hypersensitivity phenotype. Experimental studies particularly point to interpersonal threat hypersensitivity in individuals with BPD. **(p. 490)**

23.2   Research studies have demonstrated that unresolved attachment in BPD has a positive relation to activation in which of the following areas of the brain in response to adult attachment projective images?

   A. Amygdala and hippocampus.
   B. Visual cortex.
   C. Auditory cortex.
   D. Frontal lobe.
   E. Occipital lobe.

The correct response is option A: Amygdala and hippocampus.

In response to their attachment needs, individuals with BPD show hyperreactivity to socially negative, potentially threatening, and even neutral stimuli in a neural network of the brain that has been implicated in aversion, withdrawal, and even defense responses (Vrticka and Vuilleumier 2012). Buchheim et al. (2006) reported a positive relation between unresolved attachment and activation in both the amygdala and hippocampus, in response to traumatic adult attachment projective images. The visual cortex and auditory cortex are not involved in attachment (options B, C). The frontal and occipital lobes are also not involved in the circuitry of emotion (options D, E). **(p. 490)**

23.3 *Cognitive empathy*, the capacity to take the perspective of another person, and *affective empathy*, the ability to label one's own emotion in the context of emotionally charged situations, have been studied using various research methodologies. In comparison with healthy subjects, cognitive and affective empathy are found at what level in patients with BPD?

   A. Cognitive empathy is consistently lower.
   B. Affective empathy is consistently lower.
   C. Both types of empathy are lower.
   D. Both types of empathy are higher.
   E. Both types of empathy are the same.

The correct response is option A: Cognitive empathy is consistently lower.

Neurobiological data support the model that cognitive and affective empathy are distinct phenomena that rely on different neurocognitive circuits (Singer 2006). In a functional magnetic resonance imaging study using the Multifaceted Empathy Task, Dziobek et al. (2011) found that individuals with BPD exhibited worse performance than healthy control subjects more consistently in cognitive empathy and affective empathy. However, the findings on affective empathy were more mixed depending on the methodology used. **(pp. 492–493)**

23.4 What is the phenomenon called when a person with BPD is affected by his or her own emotions that are triggered through the emotions of others?

   A. Emotional triggering.
   B. Emotional contagion.
   C. Projective identification.
   D. Regressive identity.
   E. Reaction formation.

The correct response is option B: Emotional contagion.

Sharing emotions of others without self-awareness corresponds to the phenomenon of *emotional contagion*, which is not based on the proper discrimination between one's feelings and those of others. Emotional triggering and regressive identity are not terms (options A, C). Projective identification is seeing oneself in others (option C). Reaction formation is a defense mechanism, in which people take on the opposite action to an identified source of distress (option E). **(p. 494)**

23.5   Which of the following hormones plays a critical role in intimate relationships as well as most meaningful interpersonal relationships?

A. Thyroxine.
B. Estrogen.
C. Testosterone.
D. Oxytocin.
E. Epinephrine.

The correct response is option D: Oxytocin.

Oxytocin, the so-called prosocial hormone, plays a critical role in intimate relationships such as parenting and romantic relationships; oxytocin may also, to some degree, play a role in most meaningful interpersonal relationships. The other hormones (options A, B, C, E) have no role in social function. Thyroxine impacts the body's metabolism; estrogen facilitates female sexual development; testosterone facilitates male sexual development; epinephrine increases heart rate, muscle strength, and blood pressure. **(p. 496)**

23.6   Which of the following hormones or neurotransmitters has been found in reduced concentrations in blood samples from women with BPD?

A. Progesterone.
B. Estrogen.
C. Oxytocin.
D. Norepinephrine.
E. Epinephrine.

The correct response is option C: Oxytocin.

Oxytocin studies in individuals with BPD suggest reduced oxytocin concentrations in blood samples, even after controlling for estrogen, progesterone, and contraceptive intake (Bertsch et al. 2013). Although estrogen and progesterone (options A, B) affect oxytocin levels, oxytocin has the primary impact in social encounters. Norepinephrine and epinephrine (options D, E) are not involved in affect regulation. **(p. 497)**

23.7   Patients with BPD often invoke which of the following type of actions in order to achieve quick release from aversive inner tension?

A. Yelling.
B. Sobbing.

C. Lying.
D. Crying.
E. Cutting.

The correct response is option E: Cutting.

Nonsuicidal self-injury (NSSI) is frequent in patients with BPD and involves phenomena such as cutting, burning, and head banging. These behaviors can usually be relatively clearly distinguished from suicidal behavior (Nock 2009). Release from aversive inner tension by NSSI can be understood as a dysfunctional coping mechanism of patients with BPD when they try to regulate emotions (Favazza 1989; Paris 1995). Options A, B, C, and D are not considered to be NSSI, but they are behaviors seen in patients with BPD. **(p. 498)**

23.8   In addition to achieving quick release from inner tension, patients with BPD also utilize NSSI to help them accomplish which of the following?

A. Express anxiety and despair.
B. Punish their family and others.
C. Avoid feeling physical pain.
D. Terminate symptoms of dissociation.
E. Act on suicidal feelings.

The correct response is option D: Terminate symptoms of dissociation.

"Tension release" (Herpertz 1995) and relief or escape from emotions (Brown et al. 2002; Chapman et al. 2006; Kleindienst et al. 2008) are thought to be the predominant motives for NSSI, although several studies revealed that motives of NSSI in patients with BPD are complex and cannot be easily reduced to a single reason. NSSI is also used to terminate symptoms of dissociation such as derealization and depersonalization. Further motives comprise self-punishment, feeling physical pain, reducing anxiety and despair, emotion generation, controlling others, distraction, and preventing oneself from acting on suicidal feelings (Brown et al. 2002; Favazza 1989; Shearer 1994; Osuch et al. 1999). **(p. 498)**

23.9   Reduction in pain sensitivity in individuals with BPD is an alteration of which pain-processing aspect?

A. Subjective.
B. Affective.
C. Sensory.
D. Spatial.
E. Temporal.

The correct response is option B: Affective.

Reduction of pain sensitivity is not related to a disturbance of the sensory-discriminative component of pain processing but rather to an alteration of affective pain processing (Cardenas-Morales et al. 2011; Schmahl et al. 2004). Spatial discrimination of laser pain stimuli is not disturbed in spite of reduced subjective pain perception (Schmahl et al. 2004). Subjective and temporal (options A, E) are not pain-processing pathways. Sensory and spatial pain processing (options C, D) are not affected. **(p. 499)**

23.10 Patients with dissociative identity disorder demonstrate which of the following neurobiological characteristics?

A. Increased P300 amplitudes.
B. Normal cortical excitability.
C. Normal magnetoencephalography-measured brain waves.
D. Increased pain sensitivity.
E. Reduced volumes of hippocampus and amygdala.

The correct response is option E: Reduced volumes of hippocampus and amygdala.

Patients with dissociative identity disorder have markedly reduced volumes of the hippocampus and, particularly, the amygdala (Vermetten et al. 2006). On a neurophysiological level, reduced P300 amplitudes (option A) (Kirino 2006), altered magnetoencephalography-measured brain waves (option C) (Ray et al. 2006), and altered cortical excitability (option B) (Spitzer et al. 2004) have been associated with dissociative experiences in patients and healthy control subjects but not in patients with dissociative identity disorder. In several studies, dissociation has also been associated with decreased pain sensitivity (option D) (Ludascher et al. 2007, 2010). **(p. 501)**

References

Bertsch K, Schmidinger I, Neumann I, et al: Reduced plasma oxytocin levels in female patients with borderline personality disorder. Horm Behav 63:424–429, 2013 23201337

Brown MZ, Comtois KA, Lineham MM: Reasons for suicide attempts and nonsuicidal self-injury in women with borderline personality disorder. J Abnorm Psychol 111:198–202, 2002 11866174

Buchheim A, Erk S, George C, et al: Measuring attachment representation in an fMRI environment: a pilot study. Psychopathology 39:144–152, 2006 16531690

Cardenas-Morales L, Fladung AK, Kammer T, et al: Exploring the affective component of pain perception during aversive stimulation in borderline personality disorder. Psychiatry Res 186:458–460, 2011 20826000

Chapman AL, Gratz KL, Brown MZ: Solving the puzzle of deliberate self-harm: the experiential avoidance model. Behav Res Ther 44:371–394, 2006 16446150

Dziobek I, Preissler S, Grozdanovic Z, et al: Neuronal correlates of altered empathy and social cognition in borderline personality disorder. Neuroimage 57:539–548, 2011 21586330

Favazza AR: Why patients mutilate themselves. Hosp Community Psychiatry 40:137–145, 1989 2644160

Gunderson JG, Bateman A, Kernberg O: Alternative perspectives on psychodynamic psychotherapy of borderline personality disorder: the case of "Ellen." Am J Psychiatry 164:1333–1339, 2007 17728417

Herpertz S: Self-injurious behavior. Psychopathological and nosological characteristics in subtypes of self-injurers. Acta Psychiatr Scand 91:57–68, 1995 7754789

Kirino E: P300 is attenuated during dissociative episodes. J Nerv Ment Dis 194:83–90, 2006 16477185

Kleindienst N, Bohus M, Ludascher P, et al: Motives for nonsuicidal self-injury among women with borderline personality disorder. J Nerv Ment Dis 196:230–236, 2008 18340259

Ludascher P, Bohus M, Lieb K, et al: Elevated pain thresholds correlate with dissociation and aversive arousal in patients with borderline personality disorder. Psychiatry Res 149:291–296, 2007 17126914

Ludascher P, Valerius G, Stiglmayr C, et al: Pain sensitivity and neural processing during dissociative states in patients with borderline personality disorder with and without comorbid posttraumatic stress disorder: a pilot study. J Psychiatry Neurosci 35:177–184, 2010 20420768

Nock MK: Why do people hurt themselves? New insights into the nature and functions of self-injury. Curr Dir Psychol Sci 18:78–83, 2009 20161092

Osuch EA, Noll JG, Putnam FW: The motivations for self-injury in psychiatric inpatients. Psychiatry 62:334–346, 1999 10693230

Paris J: Understanding self-mutilation in borderline personality disorder. Harv Rev Psychiatry 13:179–185, 1995 16020029

Ray WJ, Odenwald M, Neuner F, et al: Decoupling neural networks from reality: dissociative experiences in torture victims are reflected in abnormal brain waves in left frontal cortex. Psychol Science 17:825–829, 2006 17100779

Schmahl C, Greffrath W, Baumgartner U, et al: Differential nociceptive deficits in patients with borderline personality disorder and self-injurious behavior: laser-evoked potentials, spatial discrimination of noxious stimuli, and pain ratings. Pain 110:470–479, 2004 15275800

Shearer SL: Dissociative phenomena in women with borderline personality disorder. Am J Psychiatry 151:1324–1328, 1994 8067488

Singer T: The neuronal basis and ontogeny of empathy and mind reading: review of literature and implications for future research. Neurosci Biobehav Rev 30:855–863, 2006 16904182

Spitzer C, Willert C, Grabe HJ, et al: Dissociation, hemispheric asymmetry, and dysfunction of hemispheric interaction: a transcranial magnetic stimulation approach. J Neuropsychiatry Clin Neurosci 16:163–169, 2004 15260367

Vermetten E, Schmahl C, Lindner S, et al: Hippocampal and amygdalar volumes in dissociative identity disorder. Am J Psychiatry 163:630–636, 2006 16585437

Vrticka P, Vuilleumier P: Neuroscience of human social interactions and adult attachment style. Front Hum Neurosci 6:212, 2012 22822396

C H A P T E R   2 4

An Alternative Model for Personality Disorders

DSM-5 Section III and Beyond

24.1 Which of the following is the most reasonable critique of the approach taken by DSM-III and DSM-IV to the diagnosis of personality disorders (PDs)?

A. The disorders have too little overlap, not allowing for multiple diagnoses.
B. The criteria allow for the possibility for a wide variety of presentations of the same disorder.
C. The thresholds between normal and pathological were arbitrary.
D. The diagnoses are so rigid as to not allow for symptomatic changes over time.
E. The diagnoses are overinclusive, leaving little room for unique pathological presentations.

The correct response is option C: The thresholds between normal and pathological were arbitrary.

DSM-III and the subsequent editions chose to use a categorical approach to diagnosis as a way to keep the diagnoses consistent with other diagnoses. Critiques of this approach occurred soon after the publication of the manual. Critiques included the fact that there is a great deal of overlap between the diagnoses such that many patients receive more than one diagnosis (option A); there is great heterogeneity among patients with the same disorder such that two patients with the same disorder can have very different presentations (option B); there is temporal instability of diagnoses such that patients may or may not be diagnosed at different times (option D); there is an arbitrary threshold between normal and pathological with little empirical basis to justify this threshold; and there is poor coverage of the possible personality types such that many specific PD presentations are not covered by the specific diagnoses (option E) (although they meet the general criteria for PDs). **(pp. 511–512)**

24.2 Which of the following explanations is suggested by this observation? The DSM-IV diagnosis of PD not otherwise specified (PDNOS) in DSM-IV-TR is the most commonly diagnosed PD.

A. The diagnoses inadequately cover the possible range of personality pathology.

B. The diagnoses as written are not reliable.

C. The diagnoses are too confusing for most clinicians to use.

D. The diagnoses lack empirical research supporting their validity.

E. PDs cannot be diagnosed using a categorical approach.

The correct response is option A: The diagnoses inadequately cover the possible range of personality pathology.

The categorical approach to personality diagnosis has a number of advantages, including its general utility, good interrater reliability, and relative simplicity in clinical practice (options B, C, E). In addition, there is empirical support for at least some of the diagnoses (option D). There are a number of critiques of this approach. One example of the limits of the categorical approach is the reported overuse of the PDNOS diagnosis, suggesting that there is poor coverage of personality pathology such that clinicians have to resort to a "waste basket" diagnosis. **(pp. 511–512)**

24.3 Which of the following best characterizes the DSM-5 "alternative" attempt in Section III, "Emerging Measures and Models" (American Psychiatric Association 2013), to incorporate both dimensional and categorical elements in the PD diagnoses?

A. Hybrid.

B. Polythetic.

C. Monothetic.

D. Categorical.

E. Dimensional.

The correct response is option A: Hybrid.

The DSM-5 Personality and Personality Disorders Work Group created an alternative model for PDs. It was placed in DSM-5 Section III. This model attempts to strike a balance between categorical and dimensional approaches, using a hybrid of the two. It also preserves some of the polythetic approach of the manual, in that a patient could have more than one possible combination of symptoms to meet criteria for the disorder (as opposed to a monothetic classification, in which the criteria listed are both necessary and sufficient to identify the disorder). **(pp. 512–513)**

24.4 In the DSM-5 alternative model for PDs, there are new general criteria for the disorders and pathological personality traits and specific criteria for each individual diagnosis. Which of the following are patients required to demonstrate?

A. Criteria for one of 10 possible PDs.

B. Impairment in personality functioning.

C. Evidence for childhood precursors of their disorder.

D. Comorbidity with an Axis I disorder.

E. Such primitive defenses as splitting or projective identification.

The correct response is option B: Impairment in personality functioning.

The alternative model for PDs in DSM-5 Section III consists of assessments of the following: 1) new general criteria for PDs, 2) impairment in personality functioning, 3) pathological personality traits, and 4) criteria for six specific PDs. The first three are required, whereas patients do not necessarily have to meet criteria for a specific disorder. Only six of the DSM-IV-TR PDs were retained, because they had the most extensive empirical evidence. Also, unlike DSM-IV-TR, the requirement for a childhood conduct disorder as a precursor for antisocial PD was eliminated. **(pp. 512–513, 526, 531)**

24.5   DSM-IV-TR general criteria for PDs described an enduring pattern of inner experience and behavior that is potentially manifest by affectivity, interpersonal functioning, impulse control, and/or which of the following?

   A. Cognition.
   B. Pathological personality traits.
   C. Disturbances in identity.
   D. Difficulties with self-direction.
   E. Lack of capacity for intimacy.

The correct response is option A: Cognition.

The DSM-IV-TR general criteria for a PD describe an enduring pattern of inner experience and behavior that is manifest by deficits in two or more of the following areas: cognition, affectivity, interpersonal functioning, and impulse control. These general criteria caused some confusion because they were not empirically validated and were, at times, inconsistent with some of the specific criteria. DSM-IV PD criteria are heavily oriented toward self and interpersonal difficulties. In the DSM-IV general criteria for a personality disorder, the cognition area under Criterion A gives "ways of perceiving and interpreting self, other people, and events" as a definition. It is also of note that although listed in the general criteria, there are few examples of cognitive deficits included among the criteria for specific disorders, which are weighted toward self and interpersonal difficulties. Options C, D, and E describe criteria for specific personality disorders, and DSM-IV-TR did not provide a comprehensive set of maladaptive personality traits for the criteria of PDs. (option B) **(pp. 513–514, 518)**

24.6   Which of the following has been found to distinguish avoidant PD from social phobia?

   A. More problems with self-esteem.
   B. Persistent difficulties in social situations.
   C. Inability to perform certain tasks (i.e., eating) in public venues.
   D. Lack of response to behavioral interventions.
   E. Greater likelihood of assigning negative attributes and emotions to others.

The correct response is option A: More problems with self-esteem.

The overlap between DSM-IV-TR–defined avoidant PD and social phobia has always been of concern. Some studies suggest that patients with avoidant PD can be distinguished from patients with social phobia on the basis of more problems with self-esteem, identity, and relationships. Both disorders share a discomfort with social situations (option B), and social phobia is defined by the difficulty persons have performing certain tasks (option C). Both disorders can benefit from behavioral interventions (option D). The tendency to assign negative attributes to others is a characteristic of the borderline PD (option E). **(p. 514)**

24.7 The DSM-5 Section III model for personality traits was derived from which of the following models of personality?

A. Eysenck's three-factor model.
B. Costa and Widiger's five-factor model.
C. Zukerman and Kulman's alternative five model.
D. Hippocrates's four temperaments.
E. Myers Briggs Type Indicator.

The correct response is option B: Costa and Widiger's five-factor model.

The DSM-5 Section III model provides a set of 25 maladaptive traits based on the five-factor model of personality traits developed by (among others) Costa and McCrea (1992) and Costa and Widiger (2002). Options A, C, D, and E are a reminder that we have sought to understand the essence of personality types since ancient times and that there are alternative models. The five-factor model remains well established and simple to comprehend, and it was easily adaptable to the DSM approach to diagnosis. **(p. 519)**

24.8 The DSM-5 Section III model describes higher-order trait domains and facets for each domain. The two higher-order trait domains most relevant to antisocial PD are Disinhibition and which of the following domains?

A. Negative affectivity.
B. Detachment.
C. Antagonism.
D. Psychoticism.
E. Neuroticism.

The correct response is option C: Antagonism.

The DSM-5 Section III model adapts the five-factor model by emphasizing the more pathological end of the domains; thus the major domains in DSM-5 Section III are Negative Affectivity, Detachment, Antagonism, Disinhibition, and Psychoticism. These are then subdivided into "facets." The section then provides descriptions of each of the six PDs deemed to be empirically validated based on these domains and facets. The definition of antisocial PD contained four trait facets within the domain of Antagonism and three facets within the domain of Disinhibition. **(pp. 519–520)**

24.9 The DSM-5 Section III model description for borderline personality disorder (BPD) and antisocial PD overlap for which of the following trait facets?

A. Hostility.
B. Manipulativeness.
C. Deceitfulness.
D. Callousness.
E. Grandiosity.

The correct response is option A: Hostility.

There is considerable overlap between the diagnoses of BPD and antisocial PD. In the DSM-5 Section III model, they have three facets in common: hostility, impulsivity, and risk taking (see Table 24–2 provided below). **(pp. 521–522)**

Assignment of 25 trait facets to DSM-5 personality disorders

Trait domains/facets	Personality disorders					
	ASPD	AVPD	BPD	NPD	OCPD	STPD
Negative Affectivity (vs. Emotional Stability)						
Emotional lability			X			
Anxiousness		X̲	X			
Separation insecurity			X			
Perseveration					X	
Depressivity			X			
Detachment (vs. Extraversion)						
Withdrawal		X̲				X̲
Intimacy avoidance		X̲			X̲	
Anhedonia		X				
Restricted affectivity					X̲	X̲
Suspiciousness						X
Antagonism (vs. Agreeableness)						
Manipulativeness	X					
Deceitfulness	X					
Grandiosity				X		
Attention seeking				X		
Callousness	X					
Hostility	X̲		X̲			
Disinhibition (vs. Conscientiousness)						
Irresponsibility	X					

Assignment of 25 trait facets to DSM-5 personality disorders *(continued)*

Trait domains/facets	Personality disorders					
	ASPD	AVPD	BPD	NPD	OCPD	STPD
Impulsivity	X̲		X̲			
Risk taking	X̲		X̲			
Rigid perfectionism (lack of)					X	
Psychoticism (vs. Lucidity)						
Unusual beliefs and experiences						X
Eccentricity						X
Cognitive and perceptual dysregulation						X

Note. Underlining indicates common facets.
ASPD=antisocial personality disorder; AVPD=avoidant personality disorder; BPD=borderline personality disorder; NPD=narcissistic personality disorder; OCPD=obsessive-compulsive personality disorder; STPD=schizotypal personality disorder.

24.10 A person who is high in neuroticism is likely to be described in which of the following ways?

A. Anxious.
B. Oriented toward others.
C. Introverted.
D. Eschewing novelty.
E. Disorderly.

The correct response is option A: Anxious.

In the five-factor model, *neuroticism* is the tendency to experience negative emotions, such as anger, anxiety, or depression. As used in the DSM-5 Section III model, trait neuroticism is included under the domain of Negative Affectivity. As with the other five factors, the domains in DSM were reworded to emphasize their negative or pathological aspects. **(pp. 522–523)**

24.11 Which of the following summarizes one of the strongest arguments for using dimensional rather than categorical approaches when diagnosing PDs?

A. Categorical approaches are neither practical nor user friendly.
B. Diagnostic schemes using categorical approaches have an inherent theoretical bias.
C. Differences between normal and pathological personality are ones of degree, not kind.
D. Categorical approaches do not allow for polythetic approaches.
E. There is little interrater reliability with categorical diagnoses.

The correct response is option C: Differences between normal and pathological personality are ones of degree, not kind.

There is considerable and compelling evidence to suggest that pathological personalities differ from normal range personalities in degree rather than in kind (Eaton et al. 2011; Haslam et al. 2012). Thus although categorical diagnoses have some benefits, such as ease of use, the lack of inherent theoretical basis, the inclusion of polythetic approaches, and good interrater reliability (options A, B, D, and E), they do not reflect the continuous nature of personality types and inappropriately suggest a clear threshold between the normal and the pathological. **(p. 523)**

24.12 Which of the following PDs has the most extensive empirical evidence for validity and clinical utility?

A. Paranoid PD.
B. Schizoid PD.
C. BPD.
D. Histrionic PD.
E. PDNOS.

The correct response is option C: BPD.

The DSM-5 Section III model advocated for keeping only 6 of the 10 DSM-IV PDs, on the basis of their prevalence in the community, associated functional impairment, treatment and prognostic significance, and, when available, neurobiological and genetic evidence. The six were borderline, avoidant, obsessive-compulsive, antisocial, narcissistic, and schizotypal PDs. Among these, borderline, antisocial, and schizotypal PDs have the greatest empirical validity. **(pp. 526–527)**

24.13 Which of the following PDs has the fewest empirical studies supporting their validity?

A. Antisocial PD.
B. Paranoid PD.
C. BPD.
D. Schizotypal PD.
E. Depressive PD.

The correct response is option B: Paranoid PD.

Among the DSM-IV PDs, paranoid, schizoid, and histrionic have the least empirical validity and clinical utility, and the DSM-5 Section III model recommended removing them as disorders and including their essential features among the traits. **(pp. 526–527)**

24.14 Which of the following is most typical of polythetic approaches to diagnoses?

A. Considers all members of the diagnostic group identical on all characteristics.
B. Includes broad sets of criteria that are neither necessary nor sufficient.
C. Makes a clear distinction between normal and pathological.

D. Considers symptoms on a continuum between normal and pathological.

E. Incorporates both categorical and dimensional approaches.

The correct response is option B: Includes broad sets of criteria that are neither necessary nor sufficient.

A *polythetic classification* is defined as a broad set of criteria that are neither necessary nor sufficient. Each member of the category must possess some minimal number of defining characteristics. However, no feature has to be found in each member of the category, and individual members of the class are similar but not identical (option A). As the thresholds in polythetic criteria sets are arbitrarily set, they may not adequately distinguish between the normal and pathological (option C). In contrast, *monothetic classifications* are defined as including characteristics that are both necessary and sufficient to identify members of a class, such that all members are relatively identical. These are both categorical classes (option E), which do not incorporate a continuum (option D). (**pp. 511–513**)

24.15 The DSM-5 Section III criteria differ from those of the DSM-IV in that antisocial PD can be diagnosed in the absence of which of the following?

A. A pervasive pattern of disregard for the rights of others.

B. A history of childhood conduct disorder.

C. Violation of the rights of others.

D. Age of at least 18 years.

E. Lack of remorse or indifference to hurting others.

The correct response is option B: A history of childhood conduct disorder.

The DSM-5 Section III model chose to eliminate the childhood conduct disorder requirement for antisocial PD. This is because of its reliance on retrospective recall or prior records to establish a diagnosis, both of which could be flawed or inaccurate, as well as evidence that suggests antisocial PD can occur in individuals with no history of childhood conduct disorder. Options A, C, D, and E are criteria for antisocial PD. (**pp. 530–531**)

24.16 In the DSM-5 Section III, diagnosis of personality disorder–trait specified (PD-TS) differs from PDNOS in that it requires which of the following?

A. The individual must meet the general criteria for a PD.

B. The individual cannot meet the criteria for any specific PD.

C. The individual's symptoms are consistent with a specific pattern of symptoms not included among the accepted PDs.

D. The specific maladaptive traits should be listed as part of the diagnosis.

E. The individual meets criteria for more than one PD.

The correct response is option D: The specific maladaptive traits should be listed as part of the diagnosis.

In the DSM-5 Section III, the new diagnosis of PD-TS is an attempt to create a category of personality diagnosis that is more clinically useful than the DSM-IV-TR PDNOS in that it includes a set of maladaptive traits to select from as well as a way of assigning a specific level of impairment. As with DSM-IV-TR, the individual must meet the general criteria for a PD (option A). It can be used when an individual has a PD that does not meet the criteria for a specific PD (option B), when an individual has a PD that is not included in DSM-5 (e.g., depressive or passive-aggressive PDs) (option C), or when individuals have such extensive personality pathology that they meet criteria for several of the specific diagnoses (option E). **(pp. 531–532)**

24.17 Schizotypal PD differs from the other DSM-5 Section III disorders in that it includes dysfunction in which of the following domains?

A. Negative Affectivity.
B. Detachment.
C. Antagonism.
D. Disinhibition versus compulsivity.
E. Psychoticism.

The correct response is option E: Psychoticism.

The schizotypal PD includes possible dysfunction in the domains of Negative Affectivity (option A), Detachment (option B), and Psychoticism. The first two are shared with other disorders; however, the domain of Psychoticism is unique to this disorder. Antagonism and Disinhibition are domains more associated with other personality disorders (options C and D). See Table 24–2 provided above. **(p. 522)**

References

American Psychiatric Association: Diagnostic and Statistical Manual of Mental Disorders, 5th Edition. Arlington, VA, American Psychiatric Association, 2013

Costa PT Jr, McCrae RR: NEO PI-R Professional Manual (Revised NEO Personality Inventory and NEO Five-Factor Inventory). Odessa, FL, Personality Assessment Resources, 1992

Costa PT Jr, Widiger TA (eds): Personality Disorders and the Five-Factor Model of Personality, 2nd Edition. Washington, DC, American Psychological Association, 2002

Eaton NR, Krueger RF, South SC, et al: Contrasting prototypes and dimensions in the classification of personality pathology: evidence that dimensions, but not prototypes, are robust. Psychol Med 41:1151–1163, 2011 20860863

Haslam N, Holland E, Kuppens P: Categories versus dimensions in personality and psychopathology: a quantitative review of taxometric research. Psychol Med 42:903–920, 2012 21939592